SHORT STATURE
AND
HEIGHT INCREASE

SHORT STATURE and HEIGHT INCREASE

Acclaimed in
American Medical Journals

ILLINOIS MEDICAL JOURNAL:
> "Pages packed with height helps, instructions, practices . . . Answers all questions on height increasing methods and measures."

WISCONSIN MEDICAL JOURNAL:
> "There really are certain things which a small person may do to increase his size apparently."

OHIO MEDICAL JOURNAL:
> "The first book of its kind."

WESTERN JOURNAL OF SURGERY:
> "Covers completely various methods . . . for the increase of height."

CONNECTICUT STATE MEDICAL JOURNAL:
> "This book should be helpful to many and of interest to all who long to be taller."

SOUTHERN MEDICINE & SURGERY:
> "A unique book with great possibilities."

UROLOGIC & CUTANEOUS REVIEW:
> "Scientific and practical value."

ARCHIVES OF INTERNAL MEDICINE:
> "The advice . . . is sane, sensible and easy to follow."

SHORT STATURE and HEIGHT INCREASE

C. J. GERLING

NEW YORK

HARVEST HOUSE

PUBLISHED BY HARVEST HOUSE, 70 FIFTH AVENUE, NEW YORK

PRINTED IN THE UNITED STATES OF AMERICA

COPYRIGHT 1939 BY B. H. LEVINE

Foreword

UP TILL now there has not been available any reputable book on the subject of short stature and height increase. This is the first comprehensive work of its kind, and no less authoritative than comprehensive. It covers the subject completely, from its theoretical to its practical aspects, and ranges all the way from physical anthropology to commercial frauds. It should interest, therefore, every adult below average stature, particularly the man on the street, for the style is popular and intended for lay readers.

The scientific value of this work may best be appreciated by the fact that the author's approach to the whole problem is predicated on the findings of our most eminent anthropologists. Some of the scientists who are quoted are Boas, Davenport, Hrdlicka, and Riddle. Much sound advice is given here on diet, rest, glands, and other health problems in relation to growth. Parents who are concerned about the stature of their children should find the chapters on growth most helpful.

The author stresses the psychological factors of short stature because it sometimes inflicts an apparently irreparable psychic trauma. He indicates a number of ways in which acute self-consciousness may be removed. In other respects the psychological aids included here will prove of inestimable value to all short people. Not only is the information practical and to the point, but it will also help set the reader's mind at ease, a condition most important in any human deficiency.

Separate chapters are devoted to drugs, exercises, and posture. Each of these is covered thoroughly, and every possible measure included which might be of service or assistance to the reader. The chapter on drugs digests all the information available on this phase of the subject. The chapter on exercises is most detailed, with specific directions and guidance. And the chapter on posture explains how one may add an inch or more to one's height by erect carriage.

Other chapters on devices, clothes, and stature aids are equally informative and helpful. The author describes the "Pandiculator," the Sayres apparatus, the Glover halter, the "Rota" bar, and other stretching appliances. All advertised height-increasing machines, of course, are frauds, though it is not commonly known how seriously they may harm one. The sections on clothes and stature aids demonstrate how the reader can add inches by optical illusions and how he can appear taller by the proper selection of wearing apparel, specially built shoes, etc.

A careful study of this work should enable the reader who follows its recommendations to improve his appearance as well as his morale. Even without any actual gain

FOREWORD

in height, he will feel taller and look taller if he obeys the counsel offered him. For the counsel is both positive and negative. Instruction on sound body-build measures is balanced by precautionary advice on the dangers of height-increasing fads, frauds, and fallacies.

SHORT STATURE AND HEIGHT INCREASE deserves unqualified approval and a large public. It is scientifically sound, sensible in judgment, and practical in conception. Throughout this book the reader is constantly directed by rational suggestion to make the best and the most of his short stature. After reading it, he should be able to face his problem with a clear mind and, what is more valuable, learn concretely what to do about it.

EDWARD PODOLSKY, M.D.

Contents

1

Introduction

NO LESS an authority than the Bible itself queries skeptically: "Which of you by taking thought can add one cubit unto his stature?" (Matthew 6:27.) And this attitude is likely to be reflected in despairing resignation by many among the short people, particularly by the males, with the result that little thought is devoted to the correction of their lack.

Now, while we certainly are lacking in the temerity requisite to question Holy Writ, we cannot refrain from pointing out that it offers no necessary occasion for complete hopelessness. The cubit, we submit, being equivalent to eighteen inches, would indeed be rather a fantastic goal for anyone save a young boy to aim at in the matter of stature increase. For that matter, an additional eighteen inches of height would place even the average short person in the freak class. But if the short man is more moderate in his desires and can be content to think in terms of inches rather than in cubits, if he is reasonable and does not hotly insist that all results be clearly discernible in barefoot checking against a measuring stick but will be satisfied with the effect of increased stature present in his appearance rather than in his skeleton—taking thought and suiting action to it will enable the short man to do much to relieve the embarrassment he so frequently experiences when in the company of his taller friends.

We are all familiar with the legend of Procrustes, the famous robber of classical times who waylaid the unfortunate Greek travelers and, after despoiling them, insisted they spend the night in an odd-size bed into which they had to fit exactly. Were they too long, he simply lopped off such excess of their members as extended past the bed, and were they too short, he hitched on a tackle and stretched them to the required dimensions. This is probably the earliest recorded efforts at stature control and it went on without ever gaining any popularity among the common people until Theseus finally put an end to it by putting an end to Procrustes.

Fantastic as this legend appears, there are nevertheless current today some methods of stature increase that involve the same principle of forced stretching by means of various contraptions that resemble medieval torture machines. Some benefit may be worked by these measures, but they definitely are not the whole answer to the problem. Increasing the height involves a number of factors, each under the influence of a number of circum-

stances, and the successful technique of a person desiring
to be taller must take them all into balanced consideration. While much can be done to prompt a growing
child to achieve goodly proportions, it must be confessed
at the outset that the increase in actual inches possible
for the mature adult is limited. Therefore, the adult is
forced to make use of more or less indirect means for this
purpose: through better posture he can straighten out
some of his bent-over inches of height; through exercise
he can tighten up some of the lax muscles and have
them support his frame more erectly; by various devices,
high heels and the like, he can seem to be taller; and by
controlling his figure, watching the cut and design of his
clothing, and by similar means, he can set off whatever
stature he has to its best advantage. In short, while the
average man may be able to bring about some additional
growth in himself, it can rarely exceed a moderate
amount, but any man may add inches to his *apparent*
height by exercising a small amount of regular care in his
dress, bearing, and behavior. Much money is spent every
year by short men all over the world in their attempts to
overcome their deficiency, but almost everything that is
effective in this direction can easily be done by the person
himself with little or no expense. It is the purpose of the
subsequent chapters of this book to examine the features
of this problem, study the manners of remedying them,
and outline practical procedures for the use of the average person in overcoming them.

But let us first get a clearer understanding of the

INTRODUCTION

fundamental nature of the subject of stature, its factors, mechanism, implications, etc., before we pass on to the means of controlling it.

To begin with, stature is naturally intimately tied up with the matter of growth—is, in fact, one of its most obvious manifestations. Hence, no sound comprehension of the former can be achieved without some study of the latter.

Growth is one of the most complex processes of the body. Stature is only one of its manners of evidencing itself; it also accounts for general bodily development. Through a process known as *differentiation*, growth proceeds along a controlled inequality in various directions throughout the body and thus produces shape. Were it not for this we should grow as a ball, the initial egg being spherical. Growth proceeds sporadically at need after one's maturity is attained in order to repair injuries to the body. When growth becomes disordered we have such things as warts, wens, cancer, tumors, etc. When growth is not properly controlled there result giants, dwarfs, or very fat or very thin people. When differentiation becomes unbalanced, we have any of a large variety of monstrosities or deformities—persons with extra heads, limbs, organs, or with some parts missing or badly out of their normal shape and size. Growth, to repeat, is a complex process, and stature is but one of its aspects. The mechanism of and factors influencing growth will be more fully taken up in chapter 4.

A good stature has been admired and held a desirable

INTRODUCTION

quality in a man in almost all ages and climes, often out
of all proportion to its real value. Havelock Ellis points
out that stature is one of the two most obvious features
of sexual attraction and selection, the other being com-
plexion. One instinctively pictures his or her ideal as
either tall or short, light or dark. It is a common belief
that the tall are generally attracted to the short and the
short to the tall, responding to what is often termed the
"charm of disparity," but actual observation shows this
belief to be far from universally true. The fact seems
to be that in the majority of instances a premium is
placed by both men and women on tallness in their
choice, regardless of their own height, and if shortness
is ever sought it is most frequently in women. This wor-
ship of tallness may in part spring from the innate demands of human nature, the instinctive desire for a
strong, capable mate, but it has indubitably been augmented by much favorable publicity received through
the ages. Almost every literary hero, from old legends to
contemporary novels (especially those by female writers),
has been a six-footer or better, and the large man has
been equally lauded and admired in many other phases
of life.

It may simply be a matter of the big man being the
more noticeable in a crowd and therefore getting
more attention. But whatever its basis and whatever its
justice there is a definite, general admiration of stature
in men, and the wise man will set himself off to his best
possible advantage in this respect. It is the first quality

that a stranger notes in one, and it governs his later impressions in other directions. It is generally taken, though unreliably, as an indication of one's state of health and robustness. It is always a bid for the respect and serious consideration of others and may prove the deciding factor between success and failure in an enterprise or in one's career.

There are various notions current regarding tall men, many of which have no factual basis. Tall men are thought of as being always competent and aggressive in any situation, whereas they are often stumbling, clumsy, and hesitating in the face of a real crisis. They are commonly accepted as having the most fiery erotic temperaments, whereas actual data show the short, thickset man to be the most ardent lover. And intellectual prowess is frequently assumed to accompany unusual height, whereas in fact it is found about as often in short men.

The relationship between intellectual powers and stature forms an interesting study. There are some authorities who maintain that careful investigation fails to reveal any dependable connection between physical and mental development, that brain power grows and matures more or less independently of the body, save for nutritive and similar needs. But there seems to be more evidence to the contrary. True, not by any means do all large men have minds proportionate to their bodies, but large groups of statistics show that the great majority of men of any extraordinary ability or attainments tend toward an average of almost six feet in height and 180 pounds or more in weight. Many outstanding men were good athletes in their university days. Gowin has drawn up some interesting tables comparing men in high and low positions in the same profession. Thus, he has measured and compared bishops with small-town preachers, university presidents with those of small colleges, city school superintendents with small-town principals, sales managers with salesmen, and railroad presidents with small-town station agents. He has found that the averages of the men in the higher positions exceeded those of the men in the lower positions by one to two inches in stature and by about fifteen to twenty-five pounds in weight. It is barely possible that most people subconsciously noted the frequent excellence of tall men over short, thus giving some basis for the admiration of good stature.

This relationship between mind and body is further borne out by studies of growing children. Surveys of large numbers of school children indicate the period of best physical growth also to be that of best mental growth. At any given time and in a given group of children the greatest ability is noted in the tall ones, and after these rank the children below average height.

Havelock Ellis has made rather an exhaustive study of the physical characteristics of men of genius, and he finds the above-mentioned circumstance to hold for them also. Examining the records of the men of genius or outstanding ability of some sort through the ages, he finds that the majority of them have been above average stature and that most of the remainder have been below the average, while a relatively small percentage of them were of middle, average height. In a list of 341 of the undoubted geniuses of history of which we possess records as to their dimensions, he finds 142 of them to be tall, 125 short, while only 74 are of middle height. Thus is given the lie to the popular misconception that the man of genius is inevitably small and puny. But the most interesting and pertinent point brought out by Ellis's study is the fact that the stature curve of genius runs just contrary to that of the common people. Among the ordinary population as a whole (at the time of his study), the great majority of 68 per cent is of middle height while the tall and the short amount to only 16 per cent each. Among the geniuses, however, those of medium stature account for only 22 per cent of the whole while the tall run 41 per cent and the short 37 per cent. The conclusion to be drawn is obvious: genius or extraordinary mental ability is not of necessity linked with either tallness or shortness, but rather is it a matter of divergence, in one direction or another, from the mass of common people of middle height and mediocre brain power. Set apart from the generality as the genius is in the matter of mind, it is to be expected that his body structure exhibits a corresponding variation.

It goes without saying that most can be done to encourage growth during the formative years. The wise parent will watch the diet, rest, posture, exercise, etc., of his children with this in mind, though an unfortunate

INTRODUCTION

number of them gives it no thought at all. However, even after the period of growth is past (after about 21-24 years of age), though the response to growth-stimulating measures will no longer be as great it is still possible to have them yield some gratifying results. Consequently, the mature person of inadequate height will do all he can to increase it by direct means and this result he may then further augment by the various illusory devices we shall go into later. And the importance of these methods for effecting an apparent greater stature should not be minimized. After all, there are many natural limitations (heredity, race, peculiar individual characteristics, etc.) that restrict the ultimate increase any particular person can hope to achieve, but the other devices will operate independently of these limits. Further, where it takes some time for the direct methods to become effective, the illusory methods exert their influence immediately they are applied.

So our efforts at height increase will be of two sorts: the direct measures—those which actually help to add to one's stature, and the indirect or illusory measures—those which will make one appear to be taller. The requirements in both are relatively quite simple and involve little trouble or expense. In the former, the regular practice of exercises that stretch the spine and strengthen the muscles that support the body, and attention to posture, rest, proper food, and regular habits of life will do about all that is possible in this direction. In the latter, a little intelligent care in the matter of dress, behavior,

19

INTRODUCTION

mannerisms, and the like will very appreciably supplement the improvement obtained by the direct methods. But the prime requisites for success are patience, persistence, thoroughness, and faithfulness. Little can be done in one day or in a number of scattered days; regular, unfailing application over a period of time is required. And do not look immediately for great improvement, but rather wait and look back over an interval of several months and note the difference. It takes Nature herself twenty years to make a person grow up; man can hardly hope to better her work in a mere week or two.

In order to approach the problem of stature increase intelligently, it may be well first to gain some understanding of the technical aspects of growth, its mechanism, and the factors that aid or hinder it. To this shall be devoted some of the chapters immediately following, after which we shall examine the methods for increasing height.

2

Height in Adults

STATURE, the distance from the soles of the feet to the crown of the head, is one of the most striking and obvious of human dimensions and about the most readily obtainable. Strictly speaking, it is not a single length at all, but a complex of a number of different dimensions, each often of variable significance, thus making simple stature rather an unreliable index of a person. It combines the length of the trunk (often a more significant measure of an individual, but not as easy to take), the length of the legs, the length of the neck, and the height of the head. The situation is further complicated by the fact that two of these, the trunk and leg lengths, overlap in part. All this is of great interest to the anthropologist, but ordinarily a man is estimated by his associates merely by his over-all height without any great attention being given to the value of its components. Generally speaking, however, variations of

HEIGHT IN ADULTS

stature among individuals are due for the most part to differences in leg length. Torso lengths or sitting heights exhibit far less divergence than total stature.

There are a number of factors that influence body build and development and hence stature. Among the more important of these are race, nationality, and region and climate of origin and development. Obviously, sex also plays a leading role in the matter, accounting for the great structural differences between men and women. If a man or a woman is sexually abnormal, it will usually be reflected in the build and stature. Naturally, nutrition, rest, amount and kind of activity, and living conditions during one's formative years will have a great bearing on final development. This is well illustrated by the fact that in England country children grow taller than city children, while in America the opposite is true. In English cities the crowding and congestion and inadequate nourishment of the poor inhibit the growth of the young, while in American cities the average child enjoys on the whole better living conditions than he would in the country.

In addition, there are some rather remote conditions that appear to have some influence on growth. For example, it often seems that the first-born child reaches a greater stature than those children that follow. However, this may be largely due to the increasing exhaustion of the average mother from a too rapid succession of childbirths. If the children are properly spaced the maximum stature is often reached in the third child. There is even some

HEIGHT IN ADULTS

evidence that the season of birth wields some power in the matter, children born in the summer evincing a definite tendency to grow taller and heavier than those born in winter.

Stature and rate of growth, as concerns averages for the whole of the population, of recent years have evidenced the undergoing of some rather radical alterations. Within the last half a century there seems to have been a definite increase in the rate of early growth, though eventual stature is not affected in the same degree. That is to say, growth is taking place at a more rapid rate, but for a shorter period of time. This may not be wholly desirable as there is evidence that accelerated growth brings about a premature aging.

But final stature has by no means been unaffected by this tendency. Numerous studies of the dimensions of large numbers of persons over the same period of time indicate that there has been approximately a two-inch increase in average stature during those years. In this connection, some close studies of college students have been made, since in many cases there are available the measurements of the fathers of those attending at the present day, thus making exact comparisons possible. This was done at Harvard on a large scale several years ago, the records of 1,166 fathers being checked against the measurements of their 1,461 sons. The results showed that the fathers (measured between the years 1875 and 1910) had an average height of 68.6 inches while their sons averaged 70 inches. Bowles, who conducted this study, concludes that stature has been increasing at Harvard for the past eighty years or more and that the mean annual increase has been at the rate of about a thirty-second of an inch per year.

Nor does Harvard offer the only evidence of this gain in height. Women have been subject to the same influence. Clelia Mosher's investigations of Stanford University women students indicated that their average stature has gained one inch in the past 30 years. Comparison of the records of mothers with those of their daughters at Wellesley, Vassar, Smith, and Mount Holyoke colleges demonstrates that the average stature of the mothers while students was 63.7 inches and that of the daughters is 64.8 inches, an increase in the daughters' height of 1.1 inches.

The same tendency has been noted in present-day school children: comparisons with similar age groups of just two or three decades back show an increase of one to two inches for the former group. Nor is this restricted to any country or nationality, for examination of the records of army recruits in all the major European countries points to a similar increase (one to two inches, and in instances even more) during the last fifty years. Even "Miss America" comes to the support of these figures: the queen of 1921 was 5 feet 1 inch in height and weighed 105 pounds, while in 1938 she was 5 feet 7 inches tall, weighed 128 pounds, and was more generously proportioned in every way.

Will this tendency toward increased stature continue

HEIGHT IN ADULTS

in the future? Dr. H. L. Shapiro, anthropologist of the American Museum of Natural History, thinks it will. He recently forecast that taller and more robust men will make up the population of the future. He warns, however, that there is a definite likelihood of their having much poorer teeth, and he gives no guarantee that their mental qualities will keep pace with their physical development. Bigger does not necessarily mean better, and in fact may work in just the opposite direction. One cannot help wondering what this may mean for the future of the race. Will we keep on growing bigger and more stupid, lax, and inept until some small, aggressive, alert race springs up to wipe us out? Or will our teeth become so poor eventually as to retard our nutrition with the consequent limiting of the growing process? One somehow cannot forget the lesson of the dinosaurs: they grew bigger and bigger, finding it more and more difficult to get enough food for daily sustenance, and finally died off because they had got too big to live.

Just what is responsible for this widespread height increase in civilized countries is a matter of some debate, but the probable factors in the matter are aptly summed up by Dr. L. B. Chenoweth:

"There is no definite answer to the question of what causes this [recent stature increase] to be true, but the probable causes of the increase in stature and weight of young people are better nutrition in infancy and childhood, less communicable disease, higher standards of living, and a higher degree of health intelligence among

people in general. Undoubtedly those who have con-
tributed most to this state of affairs have been physicians
(especially pediatricians), nutritionists, public health
workers and educators."

On the other hand, there are some things which, if
too much indulged in, will prevent the growing person
from attaining his normal stature. Inadequate diet is a
certain cause of subnormal height. Growth is a building
process that requires sufficient materials just as surely
as does the construction of a house. Late hours and too
little rest are probably the next greatest enemies of
growth. Too much activity, resulting in physiological
exhaustion so that there is not enough vitality present
for the growth processes, is another height-inhibiting
feature in the young. On the other hand, lack of regular,
proper exercise to promote good muscular tone is equally
a mistake. Suitable corrective exercises will be found in
chapter 11. Finally, an incorrect, sloppy posture not only
retards full growth, but also minimizes one's height. A
correct carriage, in which all one's height is erectly extended instead of being doubled over, will immediately
add inches to one's stature.

The question naturally arises as to what could be considered a normal stature for the average person. This
appears to be subject to a number of variations in accord-
ance with such factors as the time, climate, race, nationality, and the like. For example, as to climate and
locality, it may be said that one can note a fairly general
progressive decrease in average stature from the tall

HEIGHT IN ADULTS

British and Scandinavians in the north of Europe to the short Italians in the south. Colder climates seem to favor tallness and warmer ones shortness. Naturally, there are many individual variations and overlappings in these matters; racial intermixture alone would bring about a certain amount, but surprisingly enough, adherence to the averages is much closer than one would expect from the circumstances.

Ancient man was probably not the giant he is often thought to have been, Biblical reports to the contrary. A recruit for the ancient Roman cavalry and for the more important companies in the army was required to be above a minimum stature of only about 67.5 inches, and for some of the lesser companies he could have been even shorter. Consequently, the average ancient Roman could hardly have been of heroic proportions, else the military requirements would have been higher. F. G. Parsons studied about 300 thigh bones remaining from previous centuries in England, and he estimated that the height of the average midland English male of the thirteenth to fifteenth centuries was about 65.75 inches and of the female about 63 inches. The average stature of the United States male, as taken from the first million draft recruits in the last war, is 67.5 inches (oddly enough the same as the old Roman standard), but many regions and states taken separately gave averages exceeding this by an inch or more. The stature of the English male does not differ widely from this, the average for the United Kingdom being 67.66 inches. This, too, is subject to regional variation. From these brief data it would appear that the curve of stature has come down from a fairly good figure in antiquity, touched its low somewhere in the Middle Ages, rose again to a comparable good figure in the present, and is still on its way up.

Race and nationality (plus heredity, of which they are an aspect) in all likelihood count heaviest in the matter of stature. Stature averages taken of the principal races present in the United States demonstrate the rather amazing variation from the 62.2 inches of the Cochin Chinese, through the 63.8 inches of the southern Italians, the 65.4 inches of the Belgians and Bavarians, the 66.1 inches of the Dutch, the 67.3 inches of the Swedes, to the high of 68.9 inches for the Scotch, a difference of as much as 6.7 inches between persons whose discrepancy must be considered as belonging or as due mainly to race.

These averages were taken only of members of the races found in the United States and do not necessarily match closely those of their own countries. The tallest of all races seems to be the Patagonians with an average stature for the males of 73 inches. The Polynesians come next at about 69.5 inches. The English, Scotch, and Americans would probably fit in next, depending upon how their averages were taken. And the shortest of all European races are the Laplanders, who can boast an average height of only 60.7 inches. And of course there are always the Pygmy races of Africa and Asia in which the adult males are often less than four feet tall and scarcely ever grow as high as five feet.

In conclusion, let it be pointed out that just as stature (as previously mentioned) is not a simple dimension but a complex of a number of them, neither can it be considered as an invariable, exactly ascertainable measurement. It may change a bit from year to year or from season to season. For some reason, a person late in life may suddenly start to grow again for a while. And there is a definite, readily discernible daily variation in the stature of almost all persons. In many instances this may amount to as much as an inch. We are usually tallest in the morning after sleep, and we gradually shrink as the day progresses. This increase is probably due to the expansion of the cartilage between the vertebrae during sleep. Therefore, comparative measurements should always be taken at about the same time of day.

But there is a ray of hope for us in all this. Since stature seems to respond to so many influences and circumstances, intelligent control of such of them as can be managed should effect some betterment in our height.

3

Inheritance of Stature

THE PART played by heredity in an individual's stature is a debatable one. It is almost certain to exert some influence, but just what is its extent and nature is still open to question. And since it depends ultimately on several genes or fundamental hereditary units or principles rather than on a single one as do most transmissible qualities, it will have a complicated pattern and will not follow any simple rule, as the Mendelian ratio. If both parents are unusually tall their children are likely to be tall since they will lack a gene that puts an early stoppage to growth, but if the parents are both short their germ cells may or may not contain the growth-inhibiting gene and their children may be tall, short, or of middle height. If one parent is tall and the other short the picture is further complicated. All aspects of human heredity are extremely difficult, if not impossible, to study in any strictly exact manner. Most of what we know of heredity

INHERITANCE OF STATURE

we learn from animals, plants, and insects where we can control conditions and watch a large number of generations. But with human beings' constant crossings and intermixtures of strains, the mass of uncontrollable circumstances that inevitably enters, and the limited number of generations that we can survey, make the problem an almost impossible one, particularly as regards a complex characteristic like stature.

But regardless of our lack of definite knowledge on the matter, it is more than likely that the size of one's skeleton, which is the basis of stature, is at least to a degree inherited from one's forebears. However, one's parents need not necessarily be the dominant influence in this. One may be the heir in stature to some near or even remote tall or short ancestor. Characteristics such as this frequently "skip over" a number of generations. Thus, though stature may be transmissible, it is still quite possible for tall or short parents to have tall or short offspring. Since the average person's ancestry includes individuals of about all possible sizes and since there is no way of determining which one's influence will be dominant in a given conception, it may readily be seen that one may grow to almost any size without invalidating heredity as a factor in stature. The lesson to be gleaned from this is that the child of short parents need not despair of attaining a good height for he may be the unsuspecting heritor of some towering ancestor. Therefore, the young person who desires to become tall should always take care to do none of the things (as listed in the previous chapter) that will tend to inhibit and to do all the things (as described in subsequent chapters) that favor the development of any hereditary tendency he may possess toward tallness.

Now, stature is probably influenced most directly, as are general bodily development, defects, and abnormalities, by the state of the activity and secretion of certain of the endocrine glands. The matter of the glands and growth will be gone into more fully in chapter 5. Defects or disorders in these glands will naturally bring about an abnormal condition in the characteristic or function under their control. Thus, while a number of the endocrines seem to have a part in determining stature, by far the most important among them appears to be the pituitary. If this gland is overactive in a person, he will grow well beyond the usual limits and become a giant; if it is underactive, the person will remain undersize or even a dwarf. Therefore, it is possible that stature may be hereditary in a secondary manner. That is to say, it may not be transmitted directly as such, but conditions or defects of the pituitary as well as other glands may be handed down from previous generations and these will then affect the stature of the present person accordingly.

Without denying the effect of the glands on growth, Stockard expresses his conviction that the primary cause of dwarfism or retarded growth is still more fundamental and deep-seated. He advances evidence to show that this condition can be discerned far back in the early fetus, the shortness of the extremities and the peculiar typical condition of the bones being unmistakable, which condition perseveres to the adulthood of the dwarf. There is a possibility that the glandular condition of the mother may be responsible for this state of affairs. Pedigree tables also indicate that the disorder may be transmitted from the father, in which event it would be truly hereditary, since the only manner in which he could cause this effect on his offspring would be through the character of his spermatozoa.

Stockard is further dubious about the sole responsibility of the endocrine glands in dwarfism, because if they were in complete control of the situation they should affect all growing parts similarly, and this is not the case. Instead, dwarfism may be partial or isolated in certain parts of the body. The head and arms may be normal and the legs very short, or one thigh bone may be stunted and twisted while all the other long bones are unaffected, and so on. Is it possible (though not at all likely) that certain bones or tissues inherit a *sensitivity* to various glandular secretions which the others lack? All of which is not very clear or explicit, and neither is our present knowledge of the matter, but it does indicate the complex possibilities that enter into the relationship between heredity, growth, and stature.

It is probable that the child comes into the world with certain hereditary tendencies toward tallness or shortness, but that these tendencies may during his formative years be to a greater or lesser extent favored or overcome by the practices and behavior he is subject to in that period.

INHERITANCE OF STATURE

From infancy on mothers can do a good deal to encourage tallness in their children. They should be watched and cared for, of course, but they should not be coddled and pampered too much. Lap and arm nursing should be minimized; instead, the child should be allowed to kick, roll, and play on a rug on the floor or in suitable weather outdoors on the ground. Plenty of self-directed romping in the fresh air and sunshine will stretch his muscles, and then he should be permitted to sleep when and where his weariness dictates, as it is during sleep that most growth takes place. The floor is not too hard a place for a child to sleep; provisions against drafts and chills are the only precautions necessary. An overindulgent mother may be the worst enemy to a child's growth. Later, other growth-retarding influences enter a child's life. In school he is herded together with many other children in poorly ventilated and lighted rooms. He is forced to sit cramped for long hours at desks that are usually ill-adapted to his needs with the consequence that poor circulation, muscle cramping, stoop shoulders, bent spine, and flat chest are induced at a time when growth is still very susceptible to such circumstances and the young bones are yet malleable. Plenty of exercise and fresh air after school, encouragement of proper posture, an ample, balanced diet, and, above all, commodious, uncramped sleeping accommodations are things that an alert parent can do to counteract these growth-inhibiting influences.

Thus, one need not feel that he may be doomed inescapably to shortness by his ancestors. They may help or hinder his tallness, but the indications at present are that he still may do much about the matter himself. No less an authority than Dr. Franz Boas, the great American anthropologist, has recently affirmed his conviction in definite terms that heredity is not the prime factor in a person's stature, but that such things as behavior, diet, and living conditions play much more important parts. Subsequent chapters will deal with these various factors of growth.

4

Mechanism of Growth

WHILE growth is perhaps the most, or at least one of the most, fundamental and important of the life processes, there is as yet very little exact knowledge of its ultimate nature. Hypotheses we have, but little certainty. As good a definition of growth as any is that of Julian Huxley: "the self multiplication of living substance." This indicates the basic nature of growth as the increasing and accumulation of the *number* of units or cells of living tissue and not, as many are likely to believe, the swelling or increasing in *size* of the individual units. The growth processes of a mouse are essentially the same as those of an elephant. The latter is larger than the former only because its cell multiplication continues longer, goes on more rapidly, and the cell accumulation goes on to a very much greater final sum total. But the size of the individual cell unit of the elephant is no greater than that of the mouse.

MECHANISM OF GROWTH

This increase in cells that constitutes growth is accomplished by a process known as division; that is to say, new cells are not formed and added to the old ones, but each cell splits or divides into two new ones, or "daughter" cells, the original cell being entirely gone and two new ones taking its place. At first these daughter cells are smaller than the others, but they soon reach regular cell size, after which they grow no larger. When these daughter cells reach maturity they each in their turn become "parents," produce two new daughter cells, and disappear in the process. J. L. Smith describes the process of growth very aptly as "a procession of cell units in which each member in its turn disappears in producing its successors. The units increase in number as the procession moves onward. Generation succeeds generation until the tissue is formed."

As already pointed out in a previous chapter, growth is not a simple, uncomplicated process, but one which presents a number of very different aspects—all necessary to the proper development of a human being. Absolutely indispensable in the matter is the process known as differentiation, by which the cell multiplication is so controlled as to be made to go on unequally in various directions so that the characteristic shape of the growing organism is produced and maintained. Growth may evidence itself in several ways: in stature, in breadth or heaviness of build, in various types of obesity or fleshiness, etc. Growth also has certain qualitative aspects; that is, not only does the term imply an increase in bodily

37

dimensions, but it also involves various functional and organic changes and maturations that come about at certain periods of life. For example, during the period of puberty the genital organs of a growing person, which heretofore had merely grown gradually in pace with the rest of the body, suddenly undergo great development and the hitherto nonexistent reproductive functions become active. The rate of dimensional growth seems to go on very un-uniformly among different individuals, but Nature is apparently much more concerned about the functional development and holds it to a fairly close schedule in the great majority of people.

The complexity of the process of growth and human development may excellently be expressed by excerpts from an analysis of the subject by C. B. Davenport:

"Human development is a complex process or, better, combination of processes. It does not follow any one of the simple laws of growth but combines them all. In the uterus, growth proceeds in practically geometric fashion up to the moment of birth. . . . Again, in the adolescent period growth in stature or weight growth follows closely the autocatalytic [gradually and continuously accelerating] formula and the curve of increments of growth is nearly a binomial curve. . . . Finally, there are prolonged periods when growth is practically arithmetic as in the stature of girls from 6 to 10 years, or in weight of boys from 3½ to 6½ years. During this period the curve of increments is practically a horizontal line.

"As we contemplate [certain data] it is brought home

to us that in growth, from initiation to cessation at maturity, three elements are involved: (1) an underlying steady growth of the arithmetic type; (2) a tremendous acceleration of this basal growth by the intervention of special activators from fertilization of the egg in the period immediately following birth; (3) a lesser acceleration of this basal growth process by special activators that begin their work at 10 or 11 years after birth and reach a maximum of effect in the thirteenth year of the girl and the fifteenth of the boy. . . .

"There are different activators at work and they cause a differential growth of different organs. The fetal growth cycle affects particularly the increase of dimensions of the head, the length of trunk rather than its girth, the length of arm in relation to trunk or leg, the length of trunk rather than of legs. The adolescent growth cycle affects the increase in trunk length more than head height; the girth of trunk more than its length; the length of leg more than that of trunk; the length of leg more than length of arm. . . .

"The conclusion of the whole matter is that the body does not 'grow as a whole' . . . but growth of the body is the resultant of several growth-promoting internal stimuli. These act at different times and upon different organs and this is the essence of metamorphosis.

"In different races the relative activity of these stimuli is diverse, so that some races are long-legged . . . others short-legged . . . some are slender . . . others fleshy or chunky. . . . Clearly in the different growth inciting and regulating factors there are hereditary differences. All races of mankind do not undergo precisely the same degree or kind of metamorphosis."

Growth, then, is fundamentally a matter of cell multiplication guided in direction by the rather mysterious process of differentiation and regulated as to rate and location of greatest activity by various activators or special stimuli that exert their power at certain periods of life. Probably all these controls stem, in whole or in part, from the endocrine glands, mainly from those of the person himself, possibly in part from those of the mother and perhaps even to some extent from those of the father and more remote ancestors.

Though growth of the organism as a whole is gradual, the cell division by which it is accomplished is not. Division of a parent cell takes place quite suddenly and produces two daughters which reach their maturity in the space of about an hour. Naturally, all the cells of the body or of an organ do not divide at the same time nor do they repeat the process hour after hour. Were this true the body or the organ in question would double in size every hour. Only a small percentage of the cells of the body are dividing in any given hour. Of course, this percentage varies at different periods of life and in different parts and organs of the body. The cells that are not dividing are functioning, carrying on the business of actual living; those which are engaged in dividing have no time for this work. By the selection and prompting of certain cells to divide and the inhibition of others, differentiation is carried on and shape and character are given to the body and organs. When an individual's maturity is reached in adulthood growth ceases, or very nearly so. However, the cells still retain their capacity for division and the production of growth. Were this not true the repair of tissue losses through injury, disease, or even ordinary everyday attrition would be impossible and the body would gradually wear away. It is this capacity for further division which, when misdirected, is responsible for such malignant growths as tumor and cancer.

The subject of differentiation is as complex as it is interesting. It is very likely to some degree influenced by the endocrines, but there seem also to be some non-glandular hormones, or "organizers" or "formative stimuli," active in the process. It is believed by some that certain groups of cells supply these to other groups of cells during embryonic development, which process is often termed "dependent differentiation," whereas others hold that the rudimentary tissues carry within themselves all the stimuli necessary for their formative development, a concept usually labeled "self-differentiation." Since there is evidence to support all three of these views, it may be possible that differentiation is carried on by all three as factors: the endocrines, the organizers, and the self-contained stimuli.

Differentiation in growth is of two main sorts. One, the most commonly recognized and that of which we have been chiefly speaking thus far, is morphological differentiation, or that which produces shape in a member or organ. This operates largely through the control of the speed of growth in different directions. The second is histological differentiation, or the process that brings about changes in the substance or structure of the cells, which result in the different kinds of tissue that are characteristic of the various organs and portions of the body. It is this that permits us to distinguish between such things as heart, lung, muscle, and fat tissues, though all are propagated by the same process of cell division and shaped by morphological differentiation. It seems that the higher the degree of histological differentiation, the less is a tissue's ability to divide (possibly because it is too taken up with its functional work); and the more embryonic or undifferentiated a cell is, the more easily does it divide and build up tissue. Thus is explained the fact that muscular and fat tissues increase so much more rapidly than do those of the heart, liver, and similar organs.

Now growth as it concerns stature is very importantly related to the bones, especially the long bones of the body. One grows taller only as the supporting bony framework of the body is lengthened. Without this we would grow as a more or less shapeless lump of flesh, with all three dimensions approximately equal. When the bones cease to lengthen any further and become fixed or ossified, any additional great increase in height becomes impossible, though there are still manners in which stature may be added to, as we shall see. As the bones normally begin to ossify completely at the age of about 18 years, or a little later, it is obvious that any measures applied before this age will be more effective in producing a good stature than they will be later on.

At birth a child's bones are incomplete, both as to substance and structure. Great gaps are present in the skull (the fontanelles) which are not entirely filled in until about the eighteenth month. The lower jaw is merely a soft bar of cartilage which changes gradually to the strong, dense, angular bone of much different shape in adulthood. The spinal column is chiefly cartilaginous, is easily distorted, and does not have the characteristic curves that come into it later. The bones of the limbs of the new-born infant are made up largely of cartilage, and their ends (save for the lower extremity of the thigh bone) are at first composed entirely of this material. During the early months and years of the child's development, nuclei or centers of bony matter make their appearance in the central portion of the length of the bones. The only other bony matter in the central portion are the caps at the extremities of the bones. The portion between the nuclei and caps remains of a cartilaginous nature. That is why correct posture and sleeping habits are so important in the young. Their bones being so plastic, it is possible to impose a deformity on them that will be carried over into adult life as a permanent defect.

The immature bone, then, is composed as to length of a bony center separated from bony caps at either

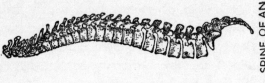

SPINE OF AN
ADULT

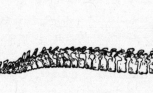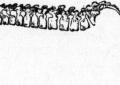

SPINE OF A
TEN-YEAR-OLD CHILD

SPINE OF A
NEW-BORN CHILD

DEVELOPMENT OF THE SPINE

extremity by sections of cartilaginous matter. This bony center between the caps is called the *diaphysis*. In the cartilage between it and the caps there arise very shortly other ossification nuclei or centers from which bony conversion of the cartilage occurs. These bony sections are known as *epiphysial plates* or *disks*. There is an increasing number of them, but they are separated from one another and from the diaphysis by layers of cartilage, often termed *epiphysial lines*. It is by means of these lines, by the increase of the cartilaginous matter there and its ossification, that the bones are enabled to grow. Finally, when maturity is reached, at about 18 to 20 years of age, there is no further cartilaginous deposit, the epiphysial lines ossify and disappear, the bones becomes continuously bony from end to end, and the possibility of growing longer so far as it is concerned is over. After that age our attempts at stature increase must seek other avenues of approach.

This period of bone lengthening is briefer in girls than in boys. In the former it is over at about 16 to 17 years of age, whereas in the latter it often is not finished until the twentieth or twenty-first year. This may account for woman's average stature being less than that of man's. After this age, it is commonly held, a person's bones are fixed as to length, and any gain in real stature he may later undergo will be due only to "interstitial accretions" by the enlarging of the cartilaginous pads between the bones of the joints and the vertebrae of the spine. However, the celebrated anthropologist Dr. Ales Hrdlicka is

MECHANISM OF GROWTH

led, after extensive investigations, to assert that there may in some cases be true growth through lengthening of the bones after this age, that a person may continue to grow in this fashion until the age of 40 or even later, and that his gain in stature during this time may amount to as much as half an inch. But even if this view is correct, the growth possible after maturity is rarely enough to make much difference to the short man and is certainly not enough to satisfy him as a solution to his problem.

Whatever may be the actual mechanism of growth, it is certain that it requires raw materials in order to do its building. This it gets, of course, from the food taken in by the individual. The matter of food and growth will be gone into more fully in chapter 6. Besides materials, the process also requires energy or motive power to drive it. This it gets in part from the foods ingested. A large part of the carbohydrates goes to supply energy, and the nitrogen of the proteins helps to produce growth of tissue and to form compounds that store some of the energy produced by the combustion of the carbohydrates and hold it for later needs. Sunlight and the oxygen of the air are necessary contributors to the energy supply. In addition to the materials and energy, growth needs certain substances that promote, stimulate, and control the process. These fall into two main classes: the hormones, or internal secretions of the endocrines, and vitamins. These shall be taken up in more detail in the next two chapters.

MECHANISM OF GROWTH

In addition to what has already been discussed, there are some less clear factors that appear to enter into and to influence growth. One of the most notable of these are the seasons of the year, though there seems to be some variance of opinion as to just which season most benefits it. One investigator, Malling-Hansen of Copenhagen, finds after studying the subject for years that there are three periods of growth during the year: from about the end of November to the end of March growth, both as to height and weight, goes on at a medium rate; from March and April to July and August children show a marked gain in height while weight increase reaches a minimum; finally, during the third period, from August to November and December, height increase is at its minimum and weight is taken on at a good rate. On the other hand, a survey of the U. S. Public Health Service indicates that children grow more in the fall and winter than they do in the spring and summer. The only dependable information to be gleaned from this is that the seasons do exert some influence, whatever it may be, on the rate of growth. There is evidence that even temperature changes play a part. Temperature changes for only a few days will often bring about slight variations in the rate of growth of children, a rise in temperature causing an increase and a fall in temperature a decrease.

What is accountable for the seasonal variation in growth is by no means clearly understood. It may be due to seasonal fluctuation in the activity of the endocrines. Perhaps variations at different times of the year in the kinds and "building" qualities of available foods are responsible. Experiments on animals indicate that these variations in growth rate are accompanied by changes in the iodine content of the thyroid, the spurt in seasonal growth seeming to take place between the times of the minimum and maximum iodine content of the thyroid, when it is increasing. It is possible that the same may be true of human beings, though at present there is no information on this.

We may summarize and conclude this matter by quoting from a report of a talk by Prof. J. C. Meakins of McGill University, in which he outlined the factors and conditions that will produce the best stature possible:

"Given a normal pituitary and thyroid function, with a proper supply of vitamin B, amino acids, ample food supply and physical exercise during the years between 5 and 20, the stature of a race may be increased to the optimum of Greek perfection. . . . In the environment, the most important factors [are] physical activity, the character and quality of the food supply, and the effects of parasitic and other diseases. . . . Exercise and physical training up to the twentieth year have a direct influence on stature. Comparison of various races of differing stature shows striking differences in the consumption of milk, milk products and meat to a degree that is considered to be significant. Improvement in the dietary is responsible for the increased growth of Chinese children who have migrated to Hawaii."

5

Glands and Growth

IT HAS for some time been known that the endocrine glands have an important role in the process of growth, especially in the matter of its stimulation and regulation. Though better understood today than ever before, the exact nature of the part played by each and the details of their function in it remain something of a mystery.

For the sake of clarity, it may be well to pause here to describe an endocrine gland. A gland is an organ in the body that produces a secretion that may be used by the body or some other organ for some physiological purpose or which may be excreted as waste. The ordinary glands—as the salivary glands, tear glands, etc.—are supplied with a duct or tube that carries the secretion to its destination. The endocrine glands, on the contrary, have no such duct (and hence are often termed the "ductless glands"), but empty their secretion directly into the blood or lymph streams. This secretion contains a chemical substance known as *hormone* which has the property of stimulating some certain other organ or function to activity. The blood and lymph streams receive these hormones from the endocrines, carry them about the body; the organs or tissues which need the hormones extract them from the streams and are in consequence stirred to action. These endocrines and their hormones are absolutely necessary to the health and even to the life of the body, to its proper development and balanced functioning. Should an endocrine for any reason produce too much or too little of its hormone, the organ or function it activates will as a result suffer disorder. All the life processes of the body seem to depend in some degree upon the normal balance of the secretion of one or more of the endocrines, and growth is no exception to this. But in many cases we are as yet not at all certain which of the glands govern certain processes and what their part in it is. Endocrinology is still a young science, and the near future should see great advances in it.

It goes without saying that the glands are most active in growth during the formative years, before adulthood is attained. Therefore, any attempt to aid growth through the endocrines would have the best chance of success during this period. However, marvelous discoveries are being made in this field and it may not be many years before means are found to stimulate the prematurely halted growth of a short person to continue to its proper end. But this aspect of the matter we shall consider toward the end of the chapter. Let us first examine the parts enacted by some of the endocrines in the growth process.

The endocrine having the most positive influence upon growth is the pituitary gland, in particular the anterior or forward one of its two lobes or portions. Further, this relationship was the first to be noted in the glandular basis of stature. It had been found by some early investigators that autopsy of very large persons usually revealed an enlarged and therefore overactive pituitary, and of dwarfs a shriveled or diminished one. These observations have since been checked by experiments upon animals. It was seen, for instance, that the surgical removal of the pituitary from puppies caused an immediate halt in their growth and development. Transplantation of pituitary substance back into these dwarfed animals, or the injection of pituitary extract, brought about a resumption of the inhibited growth.

The pituitary is a small gland located, in human beings, in about the center of the head just under the brain, and it has two lobes or portions, each of which has certain functions, but the anterior or forward one of which is the more important. The pituitary is probably the most vital of all the endocrines. Without it the life of the body could not long continue in any sort of normal, orderly manner. Its control of growth is only one of its many functions. It also guides the general development of the whole body and of many of its organs, prompts the maturing of the sex organs, regulates blood pressure and a number of bodily functions, even affects hair growth, and performs a host of other duties. It might very well be titled the "King of the Endocrines."

Endocrines often operate to produce their effect indirectly, as, for example, by altering metabolism in such a manner as to bring about the effect in question, or in some similar fashion. There are some endocrines that appear to have a bearing on growth in some such indirect way, but the action of the anterior pituitary seems to be direct. It accomplishes its work by means of a "growth hormone" that is present in its secretion and is delivered into the blood stream by which it is carried to the various tissues and organs needing it. The existence of this growth hormone has been fairly well proved by numerous experiments on animals. For example, normal rats were made to assume gigantic proportions by regular injection over a period of time with only the extract of the pituitaries of cattle, the extract thus obviously carrying the hormone. The growth hormone has been recognized only in recent years. Delay in its discovery was probably due in large part to the failure at first to recognize the impossibility of administering the substance by mouth, in which case the stomach merely digests it as it would any other food. It must be injected hypodermically and not go through the stomach at all in order to be effective.

Besides the direct effect on growth of the pituitary through its specific hormone, there is evidence that it has an additional indirect bearing on the process through a controlling influence over the activity of some of the other glands that also affect growth, as for example the thyroid and adrenals. It is sometimes held that normal growth is dependent, at least in part, upon proper calcium metabolism and that this function is under the guidance of the parathyroid glands and can be affected in their performance of it by disorder of the pituitary.

The exact mechanism of the action of the growth hormone is far from understood, but recent experiments indicate that it works by causing the tissues to retain nitrogen (which they get from the protein in the food supply), the element most needed by tissues for the building and growing process.

Strangely enough, the production of growth hormone evidently goes on at about the same rate before and after adulthood is reached and growth ceases. Extracting the pituitaries of mature cattle yields about as much of the hormone as does extracting those of growing calves. It seems that the health and function of the body is in some manner dependent upon the continued production of the growth hormone, but in what way this is true is still obscure. Among other things, it is probably needed to stimulate the tissues to repair themselves after injury and daily wear and tear have carried away parts of them.

But whatever may be the exact nature of its whole function and mechanism, certain it is that overactivity of the pituitary is commonly associated with excessive growth and tall stature or giantism, and its underactivity with deficient growth and small stature or dwarfism. Overactivity of the pituitary may be the result merely of its being congenitally too large and copious in the production of its secretion, the person being born with it in that condition, or there may be a tumor on it that stimulates it to work overtime. Glandular tumors are a frequent cause of excess hormone of any sort. Underactivity of the gland may be the result of congenital deficiencies, the wasting effects of certain diseases, or the like. Endocrine secretions are peculiar in that they must be just right—neither too much nor too little.

Naturally, the most notable aberrations in growth and stature from pituitary defects are seen when the disorder is present during the individual's growing years. It is then that cases of true giantism and dwarfism are produced, with extremes of stature of about eight feet or only thirty inches. If a normal-size adult's pituitary suddenly goes bad, he will not shrink or grow in stature to any remarkable degree. What we have already learned of the mechanism of growth demonstrates the impossibility of this. However, overproduction of the growth hormone in an adult will bring about a certain overgrowth by inducing a disfiguring condition known as acromegaly in which the extremities undergo considerable enlargement. This affects chiefly the hands, feet, and face, the bones and soft parts of which suffer a decided increase in volume but very little alteration in length. Giants usually exhibit acromegaly in later life. During their early years the excess of growth hormone to which they are subject produces extraordinary stature, and in their later years it brings about the enlargement of their extremities. Indeed, some scientists say that most of us tend around middle life to some degree of acromegaly in the general thickening and losing of youthful contour in our features, fingers, etc., that occurs at this period of life. This would seem to indicate that the pituitary naturally tends toward overfunction and that it is held in check and counteracted by forces that are more efficient in youth than in later life.

While the pituitary is highly important in the development and function of the body, it must never be forgotten that there are other glands that are equally necessary even though the scope of their activity may not be as broad as the pituitary's. Normal growth cannot take place unless the thyroid gland is functioning properly. *Cretinism* (a condition of greatly stunted physical deformity combined with idiocy) is due mainly to the absence or deficiency of the thyroid. African pygmies are properly a result of racial thyroid dysfunction. The thyroid is especially important in stature as it brings about lengthening rather than broadening development. C. R. Stockard, of Cornell University Medical College, says: "The thyroid is essential for growth from babyhood to maturity. Very probably the thyroid is not alone in its action, it may be affected by many other things and so may growth rate, but the point of primary importance is that the thyroid is the central body tending to control the rate of oxidation, and therefore growth rate in the individual. An active thyroid gives fast growing rapidly differentiating structures and linear rather than large lateral type individuals."

The thyroid seems to affect growth and development in certain special manners. It speeds and facilitates the process, but does not in itself appear capable of carrying the process to its proper limits; the pituitary must still exercise its control. Indeed, in many respects the thyroid has the appearance of being but an agent for the pituitary in the matter. However, agents are very necessary and their absence or deficiency can cause great upset.

There is a possibility of another effect of the thyroid on growth. It is fairly generally known that the thyroid reacts readily to its iodine supply. Goiter, a swelling of the gland, may be the result of insufficient supply of iodine. Too much iodine may overstimulate the thyroid, accelerate its oxidation function, and increase catabolism to the point of injuring health. If the supply of iodine is inadequate, the thyroid may be deficient in its functioning and growth may be retarded as a consequence.

The thyroid is a large, two-lobed gland lying in the throat in front of and to both sides of the windpipe. Situated close to the rearward surface of this gland there are a number of (usually four) small bean-shaped bodies. These are the parathyroid glands There is evidence that the parathyroids function prominently in growth and development, for it is they that in large part control the calcium-phosphorus metabolism. The place of bone development in stature has already been discussed, and the importance of the calcium-phosphorus supply for normal bone structure is common knowledge, to say nothing of its function in aiding the maintenance of proper nerve and muscle tone. There are some investigators who believe that the parathyroid function can be entirely replaced by sufficient vitamin D and proper diet. This has not yet been definitely proved, but it has been shown that persons suffering from deficient parathyroids can be greatly aided by such means.

The adrenals, sometimes called the suprarenal glands, are two endocrines perched one atop each kidney. They are made up of two different types of tissue that function more or less separately: the cortex or outer portion, and the medulla or inner portion. The adrenals are known to be important, but as yet their function is only vaguely understood. The adrenals probably secrete four hormones, two of which are known and two which have yet to be isolated. One of each of these affects growth. One of the known hormones, cortin, is definitely necessary for life and growth, and one of the hypothetical ones, the lactating or milk-producing hormone, has, if present, a growth relation. The medulla of the adrenals seems to produce no hormone that influences growth; both of those mentioned above are from the cortex.

The thymus is perhaps one of the most peculiar of the ductless glands. Its location is the central portion of the chest. It is present in fair size in the infant at birth, grows progressively larger during childhood, reaches its maximum at some variable time around puberty, and then gradually shrinks until at adulthood it is scarcely discernible. Many believe it to be the chief motivation in bringing about the changes of adolescence, but the nature and extent of its function are still far from understood. Opinions differ as to the part it plays in growth. Some hold it to be necessary; others assert it to be not indispensable. It seems to have been demonstrated, however, that it has an important bearing on blood formation and nutrition and thus indirectly on growth, as well as being concerned in the calcification of the bones.

Its exact value to human beings is still in some doubt, but experiments on rats indicate that it greatly favors their growth and development during adolescence. Thymus extract administered to successive generations of rats produced an almost unbelievable rate of growth in the final offspring, as well as hastening the onset of adolescence in the offspring. It is noteworthy that the thymus extract administrations produced little change in the rats so treated. It was their offspring that showed the astonishing acceleration of growth.

There is still less agreement concerning the function of the pineal gland, a small body in the upper part of the head. There are some diametrically opposed opinions on it. Some declare it to stimulate growth and sexual and physical maturity, while others maintain that it restrains too rapid body growth and mental and sexual development. The plain truth is that there is probably less known about the pineal than about any of the previously mentioned endocrines. Experiments on animals to determine its function have given, with different investigators, almost all possible results, but some experiments on rats appear to indicate that pineal extract will retard growth but hasten adolescence in the progeny of the treated animals. Therefore, its effect on growth, if any, could scarcely be direct.

Thus we see that there are a few of the endocrines that play indubitable and very vital roles in growth, several others that are necessary but work indirectly, and a few more whose part in the process is possible but dubious. As the years go by it may be shown that still others contribute in some degree. Even disorders in such glands as the kidneys or pancreas appear at times to inhibit growth. And there are nonglandular hormones, as some embryonic ones that originate during the prenatal uterine development and are carried over, that may also enter the picture. All of which convinces us that growth is a mysterious and highly complex process which being as yet but imperfectly studied and comprehended can be but imperfectly described and explained.

But what is of greatest practical interest to us is the use to which our knowledge of the relation between the endocrines can be put in correcting defects of growth, stature, or development. If incomplete or retarded growth is the result of the insufficient production of hormone by one or more glands, might we not remedy the matter by administering to the sufferer extracts or concentrates of the hormone he is lacking?

This method of treatment of disorders by glandular extracts, organotherapy, has wide application and in the years to come will be one of the big fields of medicine, but at present it is still in its experimental stage. In a number of cases it has met with remarkable success; in some with doubtful success; and in others with none at all.

In the treatment of retarded growth, it must be confessed that its results to date have on the whole been nothing to boast of, being uncertain and not overly consistent. Naturally, this method would have its best effect on children of backward growth, those who are still in their formative period and whose tissues and organs are still capable of stimulation to increase. There are some scattered recorded cases in which pituitary extract containing growth hormone was administered to dwarfed children, varying in age from 7 to 18 years, and was followed by increased growth. But the results were not convincing since they could not definitely be shown to have been due to the hormone. Anything from the season to a diet change might have had a part in it. Nevertheless, this mode of treatment has given very worthy promise at times and in some instances has effected remarkable improvement, particularly where combinations of pituitary and thyroid extracts have been employed.

The greatest difficulty in this matter is its practical, mechanical aspects. There is very little doubt that the proper hormones suitably introduced into the body where they are needed would give the desired results, at least partially. But it is no simple thing to extract these hormones in active, concentrated form. Some of them just will not be taken from their sources (as the pituitaries of cattle, the thyroids of sheep, etc.), others are broken down and destroyed or altered by the extraction process, and most of the rest, with a few notable exceptions, come out but reluctantly and imperfectly. Though the market is flooded with commercial preparations allegedly containing certain amounts of the active principles or hormones of almost every endocrine in the body, careful analysis shows them to have even when quite fresh but about one-third to one-tenth of the amount of the active ingredient rated on the label. Even this usually grows rapidly less as the extract ages a bit, for the keeping properties of most of them are notoriously poor. And as for the pituitary, it is still very much a question whether all its essential products are captured in its extracts. The growth hormone itself is as yet most difficult to isolate and concentrate satisfactorily. Some day this and other hormones may be crystallized and fixed in forms in which they will remain efficacious until used, or they may even be produced synthetically in large quantities. But at present both their preparation and employment remain in the experimental stage.

The very manner in which the extracts are administered in itself constitutes a problem. When they were first employed it was attempted to give them by mouth, but this, with the exception of a very few of the hormones, as that of the thyroid, met with absolutely no success for they are either digested and destroyed by the stomach or are not capable of absorption through the intestinal walls. Hypodermic injection has given much better results, though it still leaves something to be desired. In some cases there must be other ingredients incorporated in the extract to facilitate the absorption of the hormone. One of the biggest problems with injections is the regulation of the dose and its frequency so as to supply just the amount of hormone needed, not too much or too little. Recently there has been some promise of circumventing this uncertainty by a new method of "implantation" in which small tablets of glandular substance are placed in slits at different places in the skin. The slits are then sewed up. Thus, the system appears to absorb only as much of the hormone as it needs from the tablets at its leisure.

To conclude and repeat. The future of organotherapy probably holds much for the aid of children of retarded growth, and while it may be able to do something for the stunted adult, its application there seems in the nature of things limited.

6

Food and Growth

IT GOES without saying that normal growth cannot take place unless the food supplied to the growing organism is adequate in quantity and balanced in its various necessary ingredients. Food is the raw material of growth, the building blocks of which new tissue is fashioned. That is why the developing person requires so much more food than the mature adult. The latter requires food sufficient only to supply the energy for living and the matter for repairing the losses of injury and wear, whereas the former needs this plus enough to provide for his constantly increasing bulk. And that the types of food must be suitably balanced is self-evident. It is often insisted that "man cannot live by bread alone," and the same is equally true of growth. Just as a house cannot be built solely of bricks but also demands sand, lime, lumber, etc., to give a finished product, so with tissues. Hence, the keynotes of the question of food in relation to growth are: adequacy as to amount and nourishment and suitability and balance as to the elements composing the diet.

In addition to the above reasons, food is very important to growth in that it is the chief source of vitamins for a person. These, while supplying none of the actual material for tissue building, are indispensable as activators or stimulators of the different processes of growth and promote and control the absorption and placement of various of the food ingredients in the system. A deficiency in the vitamin D supply, for example, interferes greatly with the development of the bones, inhibiting their change from the soft, cartilaginous state of childhood to the firm, ossified condition of adulthood, leaving them elastic, easily distorted, and incapable of furnishing a proper, strong framework for the body. Lack of this vitamin is responsible for the disease condition known as rickets. Growth is also dependent upon a sufficient supply of vitamin B_2 and in particular vitamin A. We shall consider the vitamins affecting growth toward the end of the chapter.

The vital part played by food and growth may be estimated when it is recalled that the general increase of one to two inches in the average stature of the populace of our, and other, countries that has taken place during the last half a century is attributed in large part to the improved food supply available to the average young person. Its direct effect on growth is further indicated by the well-established seasonal variation in the growth rate of cattle which must be due mainly to a seasonal variation in the quality of the pasturage.

But strangely enough the power of food in this matter appears to be limited. A great excess of food seems incapable of adding appreciably to a person's final stature. This ultimate limit is apparently determined by a number of other factors. However, a diet greatly deficient as a whole or in any of its elements will certainly detract from one's chances of ever attaining this potential limit of his stature. Therefore, it is not mere *quantity* of food that is required to achieve one's optimum stature, but a diet that is *proper* both in its amount and in its elements. One should eat suitably to bring out in a normal manner the potential growth and stature that lie in him. It is not a thing that lends itself to overdoing. There are diets that appear to increase the *rate* of growth, if not its ultimate limit, but these seem also not to favor longevity. Too generous a diet long continued will not bring much extra stature, but as a rule only extra girth.

And, apparently, stunted stature is not the only ill effect to accrue from a persistently deficient diet. Some extensive experiments on rats indicate that continued underfeeding during the formative years seems to affect the very mechanism of growth and bring about, in addition to retarded development, a change in body proportions. Later proper feeding may tend to bring the various internal organs to normal, but the skeleton has been permanently affected and consequently not a great deal can then be done to rectify the unnatural body proportions. Another very bad feature of early underfeeding is its influencing the failure of the brain and the eyeballs to attain their normal size. Mere underweight can usually be corrected by better feeding, but these body disproportions are serious matters, respond but poorly to later corrective treatment, and affect the entire life of the individual afflicted with them. So, to repeat, of all the periods of life, greatest care should be taken that a person is adequately and properly fed *during* his growing years. The effects of underfeeding after maturity can usually be remedied by a period of overfeeding, but this is not possible when the deficiency occurs during adolescence.

The part of food in growth, as well as in the maintenance of life, has already been indicated in a general way. The carbohydrates supply energy and the nitrogen of the protein furnishes the material for tissue building. Recent experiments denote that cell multiplication, which is the basis of growth, receives its greatest nutritive stimulus from a peculiar split protein product that is elaborated from the food supply. Embryonic tissues are especially rich in this, which probably explains why growth goes on at a so much more rapid rate then than at any other period of life.

In addition to the organic energy-giving and tissue-building portions of our nutriment, which make up the bulk of our food supply, and the activator substances, the vitamins, there are a number of inorganic or mineral elements that must be present in our food, though in relatively small amounts, if life and growth are to proceed

FOOD AND GROWTH

normally. There are no less than ten of these inorganic elements that are absolutely essential to life: sodium, potassium, calcium, magnesium, phosphorus, chlorine, sulphur, iodine, iron, and copper. Fortunately there are only three of these—calcium, iron, and iodine—with which we must exercise especial care to insure their being present adequately in our diet. The rest of them will be found in sufficient quantities in any reasonable diet. But the other three cannot with impunity be left to chance. All these minerals, despite the small percentage of the total food they constitute, are essential to the life processes. They enter in the building of the bones, have a part in the composition of the blood, lymph, and other vital body fluids, and are necessary for the health and functioning of many of the glands and organs.

Although all the above listed ten elements are of definite importance, possibly the most important are the three that are likely to be inadequate unless steps are taken to prevent it. Calcium is probably the most important of all of them, especially for a growing child, and though it is the fourth most plentiful element in the earth's crust the average child's apparently nourishing diet will be deficient in it. The two best sources of calcium are milk and leafy vegetables. The average ten-year-old child will require about one gram of calcium per day, yet a fairly well-balanced diet with but a moderate amount of milk, say four ounces per day, will give him but about three-tenths of a gram of calcium. This seven-tenth-gram deficiency can be remedied by the daily addition of an extra pint of milk.

FOOD AND GROWTH

Iron is another mineral element that is likely to be lacking in the average child's diet, especially in that of a small infant's, which usually is made up largely of milk and cereal, both of which are quite deficient in iron. Iron is most richly supplied in such foods as egg yolk, liver, spinach, and other green vegetables.

The last of the three mineral elements that may be below requirements in the average diet is iodine. One effect of its deficiency is goiter. Another is the inducing of an underactivity of the thyroid, which in turn can have an inhibiting influence on growth and stature. As there is a good deal of iodine present in sea water, people living near the coast are likely to get enough of this element in their drinking water and ordinary foods due to the small amounts of it that are constantly being blown inland in the sea spray. But people who live near the center of a large continent, far from the sea, are almost certain to suffer from a lack of it. However, since iodized table salt has been put on the market, the problem has been greatly simplified as the regular use of this in our food and cooking will under ordinary circumstances counteract any diet deficiencies of iodine.

The lesson to be gleaned from all this for persons controlling the diet of growing young people is to see that, in addition to an ample, nourishing diet, there are five essential items of food around which meals should be built. First of all, there should be milk to supply calcium and protein. This should be taken in daily amounts of from a pint to a quart. Then there should be meat or

FOOD AND GROWTH

fish to supply protein; eggs for their protein, vitamins, and iron; vegetables (leafy for calcium, green for iron) and fruits to give minerals and vitamins. The remainder of the daily calorie need can be made up with cereal and sugar products. And all seasoning should be done with iodized salt to insure the iodine supply. Naturally, the same diet specifications are also necessary for the maintenance of the health of the adult.

The proper choice of diet items is further important in that upon it depends the major portion of a person's vitamin supply. The place of vitamins as activators or stimulators in growth and development has already been noted. They play vital roles in both normal growth or tissue increase and in differentiation. While vitamins seem to do little more than induce or facilitate proper growth and differentiation, taking no actual part in it themselves nor any excess of them apparently being capable of producing much extra growth above normal limits, their absence or deficiency will nevertheless bring about great retardation of development or perhaps actual deformity. Even lacks in the vitamin supply of the mother may show its effects in the offspring.

Vitamins affect various functions of the body; the ones most intimately concerned in the processes of growth are: A, B_2, and D. There may be others, but the indications for them are not clear. The effect on the bones of a lack in D, producing rickets, has already been mentioned. Experiments on pigs tend to show that a lack of A may interfere greatly with the development of the limbs. However, though the above vitamins are most closely connected with growth, and their lack will have the most devastating consequences, normal development really calls for a balance of *all* the vitamins (with the possible exception of E) if the growth-retarding "deficiency diseases" are to be avoided.

Though in view of this, talk of "growth-promoting" vitamins is rather futile, save in a relative sense; vitamin A has of late received some notoriety as the "growth vitamin" above all others. But more recent observations tend to cast some doubt on this. To be sure, its presence is imperative in the diet of a growing child. Not only will its absence interfere very much with proper growth, but it will also prevent the building up of normal anti-infective power, thus making the person very susceptible to many infections and consequent ill health. In addition it will pave the way for a severe inflammation of the eyes with subsequent ulceration and perhaps eventual blindness. But though A can be absent only with the penalty of great disturbance in growth, a deficiency of D will wreak no less dire results on a person's development, though the results may differ in type from those caused by a lack of A. The effect of D deficiency on the bony structure has already been described. Therefore, in a sense D has as much right as A to the title of "growth vitamin."

And vitamin B (in particular B_2 or G) is requisite for the proper growth of all animals. Its lack soon brings on loss of appetite, lessened secretion of the gastric and intestinal juices, and finally severe indigestion, all of which are greatly inhibitory to normal development. It was the deficiency of this vitamin that was responsible for the prevalence of beriberi in former years. So, to repeat, it is a balance of all the vitamins rather than the presence of any one vitamin that is necessary to achieve full growth.

Some of the vitamins can be manufactured by the body itself—under suitable conditions. For example, an embryo chick synthesizes its own vitamin C during its development, and the skin will form a certain amount of vitamin D under the action on it of ultraviolet rays (which constitute one of the healthful effects of sunshine).

But the great majority of vitamins we obtain from the plant world. The best sources of vitamin A are: butter, whole milk, egg yolks, cod liver oil (or better, halibut liver oil), the green parts of plants, yellow corn, carrots, sweet potatoes, pineapples, and tomatoes. Cod liver oil and halibut liver oil contain A in a very concentrated form, and this furnishes a very handy means of rectifying any A deficiency that may occur in the diet. In addition, they contain quite a good supply of vitamin D. Therefore, one of these oils should be given children as a matter of routine just to insure their adequate supply of these two vital agents.

Vitamin D facilitates the assimilation of calcium and phosphorus into the structure of the bones. The supply of these two elements may be quite ample, but if this activating agent is absent they will not get into the bones. Vitamin D is found principally in fish livers and particularly in that of the cod. Therefore, cod liver oil is its commonest source. Yeast is another source, though much inferior to the other. Milk, butter, egg yolks, and the green parts of plants also contain some vitamin D, but in amounts much too small to suffice for the needs of growing infants. Therefore, the only source of sufficient concentration for practical purposes is cod liver oil. There is also now available a synthetic product, known as viosterol, made by irradiating an extract of yeast with ultraviolet rays; it has in some preparations a vitamin D potency about 250 times that of cod liver oil. Some of the new irradiated milks also have a vitamin D content.

Vitamin B, comprising both B_1 and B_2, is most plentifully found in yeast, egg yolks, spinach, liver, and kidney. It also occurs in the bran and germ cell of cereals. Therefore, eating whole grain cereals (not the polished or white varieties) will aid in supplying this item. B_2 or G is also to be had from meat or fresh vegetables in general.

Thus, to conclude, if maximum growth is desired, diet must be chosen so as to provide an adequate supply of the energy-producing carbohydrates, the tissue-building proteins, and the bone- and fluid-forming and toning minerals. The food items must also be selected so as to include the proper amount of these vitamins to activate and facilitate the processes for which the other diet elements furnish the materials.

72

7

Sleep and Growth

SLEEP and rest resemble vitamins in that, while they in themselves can do little more than aid one in achieving the maximum growth and stature that is possible for him, a great excess past their normal, necessary amounts cannot do much in producing additional stature above this maximum. Furthermore a continued deficiency in them will most certainly work against his ever reaching the degree of bodily development that would otherwise be feasible.

Physiological processes as a whole go on much more freely and rapidly during sleeping, than during waking hours. When one is up and about, his system is much too busy supplying the energy and materials required by the stress of his activities to be able to spare much for any of the other vital processes. An ache, bruise, or ailment rarely disappears during the day. We go to bed with it in the evening and wake up in the morning improved or

SLEEP AND GROWTH

cured. The greater physiological freedom of our body during sleep has brought about its repair. Growth is before all else a physiological process and therefore requires sufficient sleep to provide time for it to proceed at a proper rate and to its normal limits.

Adequate sleep, consequently, is of utmost importance to a growing person. Since the major portion of his growth takes place then, losing regularly, say, one-third of the normal amount of sleep might cost him in the neighborhood of one-third of his stature, all other things being equal. Naturally, since growth also goes on during waking hours to some extent, the effect would not be quite this startling, but it would by no means be negligible and it would be roughly in proportion to the amount of sleep lost. The amount of sleep required varies somewhat, of course, according to the characteristics of the individual. Some thrive on an amount of sleep that would leave others weak and exhausted. But as a rule a young growing person should get an average of eight to nine hours each night, and if some of this is missed on one night it should be made up on the next. Further, the sleep should be got in a quiet, well-ventilated room and in a bed that is comfortable but rather firm and not too soft or downy and which above all is commodious enough for the person. There should be no cramping or crowding, either by small dimensions of the bed or by sleeping with too many other people in it, causing a distorted or bent posture or sleeping with muscles tensed.

Nor is sleep the whole of the matter. There should also

be adequate rest and composure during the remainder of the day. Too many young people of school and university age cram every waking hour brimful of feverish activity of one sort or another. Sports, organizations, social diversions, studies, and a multitude of other pursuits keep them under a constant physical strain and nervous tension. The result is that the physiological and nervous systems are so pressed to supply the energy for and repair the damages of this terrific pace that they are left too exhausted to fulfill their normal functions in the processes of growth. The consequence is that development and stature are greatly hindered and, if the state of affairs is long continued, permanently affected. Therefore, if young people wish to attain their best height they should be careful not only to obtain regular, restful sleep in sufficient quantities and under wholesome conditions, but also to have their days include several rest periods—although short ones—in which they relax completely and permit their system to catch up with the demands made upon it and regain its balance. Days that are too trying require much of the sleeping time for repair, thus minimizing the time when growth goes on most favorably.

Naturally, too little sleep and rest will wreak its greatest havoc with the growing person's stature. The mature adult can with greater impunity indulge certain abuses in this matter, though if he does so too long or to too great an extent, his general health will surely suffer. Though it could scarcely effect any appreciable

SLEEP AND GROWTH

diminution in the stature he has already attained, regular loss of sleep will certainly hinder any efforts he may be making to increase his height. Whatever small growth process it may be possible to induce after maturity will assuredly go on with much greater facility during sleep. We have already seen that a person is tallest on waking in the morning and becomes progressively shorter during the day, the difference between morning and evening sometimes being as much as an inch. This daily increase is due chiefly to the expansion of the cartilage in the joints and between the vertebrae of the spine. Permanent increase of this cartilaginous matter (as by exercises, stretchings, etc.) is one of the means by which some actual—rather than merely apparent—additional height may be gained. As it is evident from the daily temporary stature alteration that cartilage responds readily to sleep, any permanent increase of this matter would also be favored by the same agent.

Thus is advice in this matter very simple and without detail. Whether you be a young growing person or a mature adult, regardless of what measures you are pursuing to insure a good or better stature, be sure that adequate sleep and rest, adapted to your individual needs, is among them.

8

Age and Growth

GROWTH is such a slow process when regarded over any short period of time that it is likely to be thought of as a gradual but uniform process. However, this is far from the truth. Growth proceeds at widely differing rates and in different directions—now in girth, now in stature, etc.—at various periods of life before maturity, and at times to some extent even after maturity.

The most amazingly rapid growth is seen, of course, in the early part of the fetal life of the child, while still in the mother's womb. It is then that a person undergoes his maximum rate of increase. In a few short months a tiny, almost microscopic egg develops into an infant of five or six pounds or more. In the latter part of fetal life the rate of growth is decidedly slower than in the early part. The last two months or so will often bring only a pound or two increase.

And this holds for the rest of life. As age increases, the

rapidity of growth decreases. At the end of the first twelve months of life a baby weighs approximately three times what it did at birth. After twelve more months its weight is but four times its birth-weight. The increase of the second year has been but one-third that of the first year. And as time goes on this rate continues to decline in constantly changing proportion. The closer one gets to maturity the greater is the percentage drop in his rate of growth.

Nor is gain in stature a uniform thing. Though during childhood and adolescence there is always some increase in height taking place, the rate of this gain is rarely if ever even and regular in character, being subject to periods or cycles of acceleration or retardation. The average child measures at birth about 20 or 22 inches in length. By the end of its third year it has attained about half the stature it will reach at full growth. From the third to the twenty-first or twenty-second year it will gain the second half of its stature, and this will go on at varying rates that will keep decreasing as maturity is approached.

Sex, too, enters into the matter. Not only is the growing period of the woman briefer than that of the man, maturity coming to her at an earlier age when she has attained less stature and weight, but also the girl's rate of growth at various periods of life differs considerably from that of the boy at the same periods. Thus, at the advent of puberty girls grow much more rapidly than boys, but in the years that follow the boys overtake and pass them in stature and exhibit a faster rate of growth than they then do. After the tenth or twelfth year the girl grows more rapidly than the boy of the same age, and she goes on being both the taller and the heavier until the sixteenth or seventeenth year, at which age both sexes are of about the same weight and height. After the age of seventeen the woman ordinarily grows but little more while the man continues to develop until about the twenty-first or twenty-second year.

The general pattern of growth rate is briefly summed up as follows by Dr. Franz Boas, the dean of American anthropologists and former president of the American Association for the Advancement of Science: "It is well known that from birth on this rate [of growth] decreases until at the period of adolescence a sudden increase sets in, followed by a rapid decrease, which continues until the maximum stature is reached."

Dr. H. W. Haggard defines six main periods in the growth and development of an individual. These do not have sharply marked age limits and may vary somewhat one way or another, but are recognizable by certain characteristics peculiar to each stage. The first four periods cover the time of the actual growth of the body:

1. *Infancy.* This comprises about the first two years of life.

2. *Childhood.* This period extends from the end of infancy to the time of the appearance of the first permanent teeth, usually about the seventh year.

3. *Boyhood or girlhood.* This stage of development

extends from the end of childhood to puberty or the beginning of adolescence, which ordinarily will be from about the seventh year to the thirteenth or fourteenth.

4. *Adolescence.* This period has its start with puberty and ends in maturity, which as a rule means from about the thirteenth or fourteenth year—or perhaps somewhat earlier for girls—to about the sixteenth or seventeenth year for girls and the twenty-first or twenty-second year for boys. At the end of this period the person is an adult. The growth of his body, save perhaps in a trifling degree, is complete, and all his organs are developed and fully capable of functioning.

5. *Maturity.* In this period there is no advance or development in the body of the individual as there was in the previous four stages, and during it men and women enjoy normally the full exercise of their physical, physiological, and mental powers. Its extent is from the end of adolescence to about the forty-fifth to fiftieth year in women, that is to their menopause or change of life, and to about this age or often a little later in men.

6. *Senescence.* This period starts usually in the neighborhood of the age of 50, somewhat before or after, and during it there is a gradual falling off of the physical and mental powers, though the mind may stay active long after the body has begun to fail. It is a perfectly natural and unavoidable process that sooner or later must come to everyone—something of a reversal of the building-up stages of early life—and is nothing to concern oneself over unduly.

AGE AND GROWTH

These above periods account for general physiological and functional development as well as, if not more than, they do for ordinary growth and stature increase. As a matter of fact, it often appears that the rate of growth is more nearly a function of the stature a person has attained at any given time rather than of his age at that time. Dr. C. E. Palmer, of the United States Public Health Service, declares that the adolescent spurt of growth takes place in young people when they have reached a certain height rather than a certain age. From measurements he has made on about 2,500 school children he has deduced that this acceleration in growth begins, seemingly regardless of age, when girls have reached an average height of 50 inches and boys one of 53 inches. From the age of six, however, to the beginning of this adolescent spurt, he finds little relation between the average gain in height and the stature of the child. These observations are in substantial agreement with those of Boas, who finds that this adolescent acceleration in growth begins in boys at a stature of about 52-53 inches and continues until a height of at least 60-61 inches is attained. His conclusion is "that the adolescent acceleration and deceleration of growth in height is synchronized closely with actual height and that both the acceleration and deceleration tend to occur more particularly at certain points on the scale of height than on the scale of chronological age."

Of course, this age and rate of growth pattern is not wholly immutable. There are factors and conditions that are able to alter it. For example, glandular disorders and certain diseases can greatly disturb the relationship. The former has already been discussed in chapter 5. The latter will be gone into in the next chapter. And then there is the matter of the notable increase in average stature that has taken place in the past 50 years. This in itself proves that stature is not an invariable characteristic. And further, some recent extensive studies made in the German army and among German children seem to bear out the observation made elsewhere that there is a tendency not only toward greater stature, but also toward more rapid growth and even earlier general bodily development, as evidenced by an increasing number of children walking before the end of their first year, by the fact of dentition, both primary and secondary, taking place noticeably earlier, and by the onset of puberty occurring at an earlier age. Thus it may be seen that the limits of growth, its general rate, and its rate at various periods of life are all susceptible of alteration.

Growth, as concerns stature, is commonly thought of as being ended in a man at the age of about 21, though some estimates have admitted its possible continuance to the age of about 24. After this any actual increase in height has usually been laid to "interstitial accretions," the expansion of the cartilage in the joints and between the spinal vertebrae, but any real growth through bone lengthening has hitherto been considered impossible. However, Dr. Ales Hrdlicka, of the Smithsonian Institution, doubts this and, after making thousands of measurements to confirm his belief, asserts that it is possible for the stature of an adult gradually to increase until the age of 40. This gain in height between the ages of 24 and 40, he says, may amount to as much as one-third of an inch or better. Indeed, he further states, in some instances detectable growth in stature may be found even in the fifth and sixth decades of life. All of which tends to demonstrate that the formerly accepted age rate of growth relationship is by no means a hard and fast one.

As a matter of fact, in view of more recent and extensive data and measurements it is rather difficult to establish any reasonably close relations between stature and growth and the various factors controlling them. Perhaps there are elements in the matter not yet recognized. It may be there are too many variable factors in the situation to permit of any practical solution. At least so thinks the editor of the *Journal* of the American Medical Association who speaks thusly in this connection:

"The inherent difficulties [of establishing any close, valid relationship between age, height, and weight] seem obvious, because the relation between age, weight and height varies in different age periods and also in the same individual. The fact of the matter is that our height and weight tables do not represent actual standards but only approximate averages. With such variable data a mathematical formula would be of no value. If one attempted the solution of such a problem one would have to obtain an equation in which the weight could be expressed as a function of the height and age.

AGE AND GROWTH

Since there is no constant relation between age, height and weight, such a formula would be useless, and any results obtained would lack mathematical validity. We simply do not possess the information necessary to state the range of variations which should be regarded as normal in each case. There are many factors to be considered in height and weight for a given age, such as season, nutrition, exercise and mental activity. There are individual differences among races, as well as among children from wealthy and poor families. Therefore a mathematical expression of the relationship does not seem feasible."

While the above is doubtless quite true, there nevertheless remain some approximate relations in this matter, based on averages, that often aid in getting some estimate of an individual's degree of normality in his development. These are most conveniently expressed in the form of tables, examples of which will be found in chapter 16.

9

Disease and Growth

GROWTH, to repeat, is a physiological function into which the vital forces of the body enter and for which they are necessary. If anything affects, inhibits, or alters the balance of these forces, it is only to be expected that growth also will be interfered with. We have already seen previously, in chapter 5, what havoc can be wrought by disorders in the endocrine glands and their secretions, striking anomalies of growth and development being produced. We have also seen that improper food and insufficient sleep and rest, by upsetting the body forces and functions, can work adversely in this matter. In addition to this, there are some diseases and disease conditions which, while not in themselves closely associated with the processes of growth, can by impairing the general health, vigor, and normal functioning of the body affect growth and retard stature.

Extensive studies of U. S. Army recruits have revealed

that there is a close relation between physique and pathological defects and conditions. For example, a very large portion of those of low stature were found to have defective teeth and refractive errors of the eye. Men who suffered from tuberculosis, organic and functional diseases of the heart, and errors of refraction in the eye, were found commonly to be of small chest circumference. Those with asthma were generally of low height and of abnormally low weight. But defective and deficient teeth and congenital defects of the sexual organs were most commonly found associated with shortness, underweight, and smallness of chest. There are other relationships that may be found. In some cases the diseased condition may be regarded as the causative element in the retardation of development, while in others both the condition and the retardation appear as associated symptoms of some more fundamental affection.

Naturally, if there are such things as diseased conditions of the liver and kidney, or if there are chronic digestive disorders, growth is very likely to be disturbed. It stands to reason that anything which interferes with the assimilation of the raw materials of growth, food, or with the elimination of its waste matter is bound to exert a restraining and disordering influence on growth itself. Therefore, one of the first cares of whoever would grow tall is, in addition to the precautions given in antecedent chapters, to maintain himself in the best possible general health, to do all that can be managed to promote proper, complete, and tranquil digestion, and to keep the

DISEASE AND GROWTH

bowels and other organs of elimination clear and functioning regularly and adequately.

A disease such as diabetes, says Dr. T. Wingate Todd, director of the Brush Foundation and head of the Department of Anatomy at Western Reserve University, when present in a young child can bring about a retardation of two to four years in its bone development and consequently much affect its growth and stature. He advocates regular, consistent X-ray study of growing children as a check on the development of their skeleton and a means of discovering any defects in time to remedy them. These skeletal defects from diabetes, he asserts, respond marvelously to insulin and faithful treatment with it will generally enable a child to make good his lost progress.

Various diseases exercise a definite influence on growth in such a manner as to alter body build, certain affections being associated with certain types of build in the great majority of cases. Thus, for example, in young persons a slender build and diseases of the respiratory tract (tuberculosis, bronchitis, pneumonia, etc.), nervous diseases, and general infections such as fevers, diphtheria, typhoid, and others of this sort are frequently found associated, just as persons of a fleshy build are more likely to be afflicted with bladder and kidney trouble, apoplexy, paralysis, and similar disorders.

It is not necessarily always a straightforward, easily recognizable disease that is at the root of growth disturbance. Often it may be a hidden source of infection, as pus pockets at the tooth roots or in the tonsils, that constantly give off just enough bacteria to hinder the body's full development without producing any obvious, out-and-out disease condition. Dr. Sydney Pern puts the case very aptly:

"If we take a child with infected tonsils, it may be apparently healthy or it may be undersized, it may be backward in its classes. Apply all the known clinical methods we have at our disposal in investigating the case. You may find nothing, yet sufficient pathological changes are taking place to stunt the child's growth, bodily and mentally, and unless this infection is removed it will grow up more or less healthy, perhaps, never suffering from any definite disease, yet never strong, nothing like what it normally would have been without the infection.

"Three quarters of the population of civilized communities are growing up like this, or have been, until the last few years."

Diseases, and especially those of childhood and adolescence, are too much taken as being merely things in themselves that incur only the dangers and consequences which go with the particular illness. It is coming more and more to be realized that these affections not only have their specific results and hazards, but also have more remote and far-reaching effects, not least among which are those upon growth, stature, and general bodily development. The conscientious parent who wishes his child to reach full maturity will not dismiss any youthful ill as one of those matters that "all children have and grow out of," but will have it promptly and completely remedied. He will take any undue lag in the child's normal development as an indication of something wrong and will have it thoroughly examined by a competent physician while there is still time to correct any trouble that may be present.

While on the subject of disease and growth, it may not be amiss to spend a moment in considering that grossly misunderstood matter of "growing pains." Now, growth is a natural, normal process or function and it should never proceed to the accompaniment of pain any more than should any of the other bodily functions —digestion, urination, etc.—if they are going on healthily. When there is pain it is not "one of those things that all growing youngsters have to go through," but it may be taken as a definite indication that there is something wrong somewhere, which if not corrected may lead to more or less serious complications.

"Growing pains" have as a rule a number of general, readily recognized symptoms that the alert parent should have no difficulty in discerning. The first indication is as a rule poor appetite. This is shortly followed by general paleness and wanness. The child has little endurance, tires very easily, hasn't any or only a little interest in his usual activities, and finds his schoolwork difficult and a burden. Many times this is accompanied by headaches and vague pains in different parts of the body. At times the child's nose may bleed without any apparent cause.

This condition, it is the consensus of medical opinion,

exhibits symptoms that are the same as those that usually go with a hidden infection. They are warnings that somewhere in the child's body there is a concealed focal infection. This focal infection may be a colony of bacteria entrenched in certain tissues somewhere in the body whence are given off poisons or toxins that get into the blood stream and are carried to every part of the body, affecting the joints, muscles, nerves, heart, or any other organ or tissue, and causing fatigue, pain, and the other symptoms above mentioned.

In seeking the location of this hidden focal infection, it was found almost always to be associated with phlebitis, or inflammation of the veins, of the legs. This can usually be traced to the previous existence of certain common contagious diseases, as measles, scarlet fever, tonsillitis, bronchitis, colds, etc. During any of these sicknesses there is sluggishness in the blood circulation in the legs at which time any little exertion on the part of the patient, such as standing, produces a congestion in the legs. This congestion furnishes ideal conditions for the disease germs, carried by the blood stream, to locate there and develop their poisons which are in turn carried to all parts of the body where they may give rise to "growing pains." If the poisons attack the muscles the outcome is rheumatism; if they settle in the joints the result is arthritis; if they go to the nerves there will be sciatica or some form of neuritis; and if they go to the heart there will be inflammation of that organ. This heart condition is a serious and a quite frequent complication of "growing pains," resulting usually in permanently weakened heart muscle and leaky valves and leading often to early death.

Therefore, let parents be warned. "Growing pains" are not at all what the name implies, but are really indications of a concealed infection which if not properly attended to may well end in serious or even fatal consequences.

10

Drugs and Height

MAN is by nature both indolent and superstitious or credulous. Perhaps one of the best measures of his intelligence is the manner in and the extent to which it enables him to combat these fundamental urges. In many respects modern man has done very well in overcoming these congenital handicaps, but in the vast majority of instances he is as a child of nature in the hands of the patent medicine quack. Being lazy, man instinctively shies at the regular attention and faithful daily effort requisite to bring about any bodily improvement such as stature increase, through the normal, intelligent means of better diet, sleep, living habits, exercise, etc., preferring to dispense with the bother while gaining the benefit merely by taking some (usually expensive) pill or "elixir." Being superstitious, man believes that the pill or medicine is able to do the work.

While it appears to be true that patent-medicine frauds

in the field of stature increase are much less prevalent than they are in many other fields of human ills and defects, there are nevertheless some to be found, and *against them the reader is without reservation warned.* To be sure, some of them may do him no especial harm, though others may. But none of them will accomplish his object and all of them will waste his money and cause loss of time that might be profitably employed with measures that will effect some improvement in stature.

Now, while there are some drugs and substances that do affect the growth processes, they are not of a sort to be put into a pill that can be taken carelessly at will by the average individual and result in a sudden spurt in height. These substances are selective in their action—working only in certain directions—must be administered in special manners, and cannot merely be swallowed; the size and frequency of dosage must be carefully regulated. All in all, if these drugs have any application to practical stature increase, it certainly is a matter for a physician with specialized training and not one for self-experimentation by a layman with patent medicines.

The action of some of these growth-promoting substances is not always clear and not always desirable. For example, growth of any sort requires cell multiplication, but if this is stimulated in a wrong direction the result will be such abnormal growths as tumors or cancers rather than general body increase. A substance that seems to act in this manner is tar. It has been noticed for some time that workers around gasworks who come into contact with tar are especially likely to suffer from cancerous growths. These observations were later substantiated by experiments on animals. Painting tar on their skins was found to bring on cancer. There have been indications of other chemical substances, some of which may be isolated from tar, which when applied to the animal, either by spreading on or by injection, have the property of causing the wild cell growth that is cancer. Other agents, too, may produce cancerous growths, as the secretions of certain animal parasites, the application of extreme cold, x-radiations, and others, to say nothing of a probable large number of as yet unknown causes.

The above growth-stimulating agents are productive only of disease conditions and are therefore of no value in promoting normal growth or increasing height. Since, as we have already seen, the process of growth is pretty much under the domination of the endocrines, one of the most logical methods of influencing it would be by the administration of substances that stimulate or favor the activity of the glands in question. Thus, the most effective growth-promoting agents will not work directly on the growth process itself, but will operate indirectly by first influencing the endocrines in the proper direction and then they in turn will affect the process.

The most potent of such agents would be, naturally, the vital principle of the glands themselves, namely the hormones. The part played in growth by these substances and the effect and success of the administration of preparations or extracts of them has already been discussed in some detail in chapter 5. The activity of some of the glands concerned in growth may also be affected by certain drugs or chemicals as, for example, the thyroid which reacts very definitely to the supply of iodine the system is receiving.

Other chemical substances that exercise an influence over growth are the vitamins, those compounds which are found in various foods in tiny quantities but which have such power over a number of the body processes. The vitamins have already been treated in chapter 6.

Naturally, many of these substances that promote growth will by their absence tend to retard it. There are, however, some agents whose only effect is to inhibit growth, and these of course are to be avoided as much as possible, particularly by young, growing people. Tobacco is possibly the commonest of these. While it may be used in moderation with relative impunity by the adult, it appears not only to retard growth and development in the adolescent, but it is injurious to general health as well. This poor health in turn forms part of a vicious circle that further impedes growth by the interference with the healthful functioning of the system as a whole. There has been much debate as to just how tobacco affects growth, but it remains fairly obvious that in some manner its regular use proves deleterious. To a lesser degree, the same may be said about alcohol. Its moderate employment by the adult seems generally to be without especial bad effect, but its regular use by the growing adolescent is very likely to affect his development adversely. And, of course, narcotics as a whole, and in particular cocaine, morphine, and above all marijuana, fall very definitely into this category. These last are especially worthy of consideration, not only because they are more potent in this and other consequences, but also because their sale among young people, and even schoolchildren, has grown alarmingly in recent years.

Thus, to sum up the matter of drugs and growth: Waste no money on fake or dangerous quack patent medicines alleging to induce growth. Place most reliance in agents that work through the glands, realizing that even here their power is quite limited as yet. *Take no drug or preparation of any sort for this purpose save on the advice and prescription of a competent physician.* Do not allow faith in the power of medicine to cause you to neglect the other means of encouraging growth outlined elsewhere in this book. Usually they will prove more efficacious than the former, especially with adults who would increase their height slightly. And, finally, take care to avoid as completely as possible all growth-retarding agents and influences.

11

Exercises and Height

THE need for regular, proper exercise for the encouragement and aid of the growth processes in going on to their full limits has already been mentioned in a preceding chapter. Not only is it of value in stretching the muscles, joints, and vertebrae so as to help in gaining one's maximum stature, but it also further promotes the health and functioning of the entire body and its organs so as to permit them to grow and develop with the greatest possible facility and in the normal directions.

Exercise is of further benefit in that it tends to bring about a better, more erect carriage or posture of the body in standing and walking. Since it is obvious that one cannot have the full advantage of his stature, whatever it may be, unless he holds it uprightly and does not lose part of it by a drooping, bent-over bearing, the importance of posture improvement in height increase is readily apparent. Suitable exercise is one of the best

97

means of gaining better posture. But this matter will be taken up more fully in chapter 13.

General, all-around exercise in proper amounts, therefore, is necessary for the health and full development of the growing person. It is also beneficial for the adult, but for him there are in addition certain special forms of exercise. It is with these special stretching or "height-increasing" exercises that the present chapter is mainly concerned.

Generally speaking, height-increasing exercises are those movements that tend to stretch and strengthen the muscles that support the body and hold it erect. This stretching at the same time favors accretion of cartilaginous matter in the joints and between the spinal vertebrae which may produce some slight increase in stature. Naturally, some movements favor this more than others and we shall shortly describe several of them.

These exercises are not difficult nor do they consume much time, but their chief requisites for success are regularity, faithfulness, perseverance, and thoroughness in their practice. They should be done with precision and gusto, not limply and boredly as if performing a chore. The entire body and all its muscles should be made to participate to as great an extent as feasible. The muscles of the abdomen are not to be neglected as their tone contributes much to the proper functioning of the digestive organs which in turn have much bearing on the health of the body as a whole and on the insurance of the height-increasing measures being practiced.

EXERCISES AND HEIGHT

The exercises should be done regularly at least once daily and preferably twice. The best time to do them is usually in the morning upon arising. The body then is fresher and fuller of vitality than later, the muscles are relaxed and more impressionable, and one has the advantage of the daily stature increase gained during sleep, part of which suitable exercises may gradually enable one to retain permanently. The best time for the second session with them will probably prove to be at night before retiring. The exercise then will relax strained muscles and leave them more open to the physiological processes of repair and increase that go on best during sleep, and the stretching will give an impetus to the nightly expansion of the cartilage in the joints and thus perhaps permit it eventually to go a bit farther. The exercises should be performed in a quiet room with ample space to permit free, unhindered movement, and with a good supply of fresh air. They should be done with as little clothing on to restrict motion as is practicable. Indeed, if circumstances allow, it is good to practice them nude.

However, the value of general outdoor exercise for the person who is interested in his height must not be ignored. In addition to the special height-increasing exercises we shall outline, it is well for one to indulge regularly in one or more sports. Any activity that causes the muscles to function, remain elastic, and above all *stretch* will very much aid our purpose, Walking, running, dancing, swimming, jumping, golf, hockey, football, wrestling, or almost any of the active sports will prove of help. Gymnasium work, too, is good, particularly that involving hanging and swinging from bars or rings, climbing of ropes, etc. This general exercise will furnish a fine balancing or equalizing influence for the more specific height-increasing exercises and will be of further benefit by promoting and maintaining the general health of the entire body.

Our first attention in improving our stature should be to our breathing. If we genuinely wish to be well developed and would carry ourselves correctly and becomingly, it is obvious that we can do much by learning to breathe properly and deeply and to gain control of the diaphragm. Deep breathing is necessary for the purification of the blood so that it may build up a good quality of muscle, tissue, and bones and generally aid the processes of growth throughout the body. Also, the full expansion of the chest offers in itself an excellent means of stretching the spine and many important muscles and of encouraging a correct posture, all of which are height-increasing aids.

Deep breathing should not be regarded as a matter for occasional attention, a thing to which one devotes a five-minute period morning and evening. Rather should the *habit* of deep breathing be established so that one goes about throughout the day filling his lungs well (though not necessarily to the straining point as in breathing exercises) with each inhalation. Also, at intervals during the day a person should consciously fill his lungs to the utmost, hold them full for a few seconds, and then slowly exhale, repeating the procedure several times. This is very simple, requires no preparations or accommodations, and can be done as one goes about his daily business. This regular, habitual deep breathing will be of far more benefit than a few strenuous but scattered breathing exercises. But the exercises do help definitely and they are valuable in aiding the establishment of the habitual deep breathing and in strengthening the respiratory muscles so as to make that breathing less an effort.

BREATHING EXERCISES

1. Stand erect before an open window with the arms hanging at the sides and the head held well up. Raise the arms slowly sideways to shoulder height while inhaling deeply. Hold this position for a moment. Then, keeping the arms raised, move them backward as far as possible, dropping them just a trifle, tilt the head back, and strive to force a little more air into the lungs. Hold for a few seconds and then return to the original position while exhaling slowly. Repeat the whole exercise four or five times.

2. Stand as in the preceding exercise. Raise the arms sideways as before but time the inhalation so that the lungs are about half filled when the arms are at shoulder height. Pause here a moment, then continue the arm motion until they are upright above the head, at the

same time rising slowly on the toes and completing the inhalation to full lung capacity. Hold this posture for a short while and then return slowly to the starting point while exhaling. Repeat four times.

3. Stand as before in front of an open window. Raise the arms slowly forward to shoulder height, inhaling at the same time so that the lungs are only moderately filled, about one-third capacity. After a moment's pause, continue the arm motion until they are above the head, carrying on the inhalation to about two-thirds lung capacity. Again pause briefly and then bring the arms backward and downward to a little below shoulder level, tilting the head back and filling the lungs to their limit. Hold this pose and the breath as long as is comfortably possible, then while exhaling, return slowly to the first position. Repeat the whole routine three or four times.

Among the exercises that tend to stretch the various joints, members, and muscles, there are some that exert their effect more on certain portions of the body than upon others. Consequently, by choosing among them and stressing certain of them there can be some attempt to correct the proportions of the body. The exercises may conveniently be divided into the following groups according to the nature of their greatest effect:

I. Exercises stretching the neck and upper spine (with some effect on the shoulders and chest);
II. Exercises stretching the spine and back (with some effect on the legs);

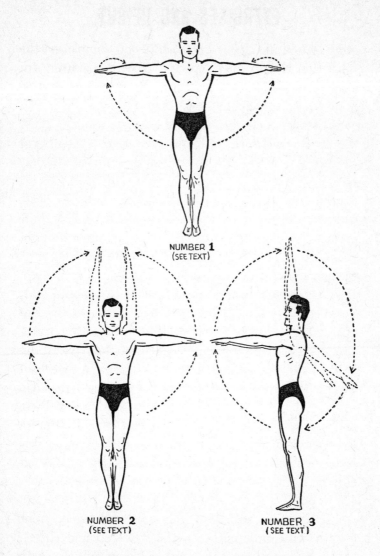

NUMBER **1**
(SEE TEXT)

NUMBER **2**
(SEE TEXT)

NUMBER **3**
(SEE TEXT)

BREATHING EXERCISES

EXERCISES AND HEIGHT

   III. Exercises stretching the abdomen and back (with
         some effect on the arms and legs);
   IV. Exercises stretching the arms, legs, and trunk;
    V. Exercises stretching the entire body.

We shall take up these categories in order, giving
several representative exercises under each heading. It
is understood, of course, that there are a number of
similar and equally effective exercises of each kind possible, but our space forces us to be content with a selection from among the better of them. These will be found
ample to work all the benefit practicable through
exercise.

I.   EXERCISES STRETCHING THE NECK AND UPPER SPINE

1. Stand in an easy, upright posture with the head up
and the shoulders back. Raise the arms and interlace
the fingers firmly behind the head, cupping the hands
about the roundness of the head to obtain good support.
Press the head forward with the hands as far as possible
until the chin almost rests upon the chest, all the while
firmly resisting the pressure of the hands with the neck
muscles. Then press the head backward as far as it will
go against the resistance of the hands. Continue this
motion alternately backward and forward, always moving
against resistance, until the neck muscles begin to grow
tired.

2. Take the same position as above with the hands

EXERCISES AND HEIGHT

behind the head. Without allowing the head to slip within the hands as they offer some resistance to the motion, twist the head as far as can be managed to the right, until the chin comes over or touches the shoulder, keeping the elbows well back. Do the same toward the left, and then alternate from side to side in rapid succession until weariness is felt.

3. Stand erect with the hands at the sides. Sweeping the forearm upward in front of the chest and face, bring the left arm straight up over the head and then (keeping it all in one smooth motion) extend it with straight elbow upwards and sideways from the shoulders at an angle of about 45° and at the same time raise the right arm sideways at about the same angle below the shoulder. Hold this position for 15 or 20 seconds while straining the arms away from each other in the directions they are pointing with all the strength possible, then return to the original position. Do the same raising the right arm, and repeat the entire routine three or four times.

II. EXERCISES STRETCHING THE SPINE AND BACK

1. Lie on the floor flat on the back with the muscles relaxed, arms at the sides. Stretch all the muscles of the back, hips, legs, and shoulders as if trying to make oneself longer, pointing the toes, arching the chest, and pressing back on the head with the effort. Relax. Repeat the effort, but this time raise the arms upward and backward until they lie on the floor past the head when the

105

greatest stretching strain occurs. Alternate these two exercises six or eight times. If the circumstances of one's surroundings permit, a very helpful variation of this exercise may be practiced by hooking the toes beneath a heavy piece of furniture so arranged that when the arms are extended over the head the hands can grasp some solid object, and the extremities, by pulling, may thus subject the entire length of the body to an additional forceful stretching.

2. Much the same exercise may readily be performed at odd moments during the day without preparation or bother and will be found of much value to office workers who are forced to sit cramped for long hours over a desk. The person merely sits as far forward as possible on the edge of his chair, leaning his shoulders against the upper part of the back and extending his legs straight before him with the heels on the floor, thus throwing the entire body into very nearly a straight line. He then stretches his body vigorously throughout its length, arching his chest, bringing his head and shoulders back, and elevating his mid-portion so that he rests against the edge of the chair with his thighs. He holds this position for a moment, keeping his muscles firmly taut, and then relaxes, repeating the maneuver several times. If circumstances allow doing so without attracting too much attention, this exercise may be augmented by raising the arms above the head while doing the stretching.

3. Sit on the floor on the right hip with the upper

body turned toward the right and both hands placed for support on the floor a bit to one side and ahead of the right hip. The right leg lies along the floor with the knee bent and the left foot is close to the right foot. The bent left knee is upright in the air. From this position stretch the left leg as straight as possible, pointing the toe, and strain the shoulders somewhat in the opposite direction by pressing on the floor with the hands, keeping most of the body's weight resting on the right hip and thigh. Hold for a few seconds, relax, then reverse the position of the body and do the same thing on the left side, stretching the right leg. Repeat these movements alternately six or eight times.

III.   EXERCISES STRETCHING THE ABDOMEN AND BACK

1. Stand with the feet about eighteen inches apart, hands on hips, head and shoulders back. Keeping the upper part of the body as straight as possible, lean it toward the right while in a smooth, uniform motion transfer the weight to the right leg and slowly raise the straight left leg as high as can be managed. Return slowly to the original position, relax, then repeat leaning toward the left. Continue this alternately until weariness is felt. If at first one has difficulty in maintaining his balance, he may help himself by grasping a chair or some other object until he becomes more expert.

2. Stand with the back against the back of a solid chair, grasping the chair's back in the rear firmly with

both hands. Thus supported, raise the right leg slowly forward, pointing the toe gradually as it comes up and taking care not to let the knee bend. Bring the leg just as high as possible, not allowing the hips to sag forward with the effort. With a little practice one should be able to bring the foot at least level with the waist. Hold the leg there for a second and then return it slowly to the floor. Repeat this three times, then do the same with the other leg, and continue alternately four or five times.

3. Sit on the floor with the legs extended straight in front. Hook the fingers beneath the thighs close to the buttocks and with this support lower the upper body slowly backward to the floor. As the body approaches the floor the hands should be released and the arms extended sideways from the shoulders along the floor. Relax in this position for a second, then tensing the muscles slowly, rise again to a sitting posture, once more hooking the fingers beneath the thighs and pulling. Finish the movement by leaning well forward and touching the toes with the fingers. Repeat the entire exercise five or six times.

IV.   EXERCISES STRETCHING THE ARMS, LEGS, AND TRUNK

1. Stand up straight with the arms at the sides. Take a full stride forward with the right leg, putting it out as far as it will go, and at the same time raise the arms sideways level with the shoulders and twist the upper body from the waist well to the right. In this position swing the

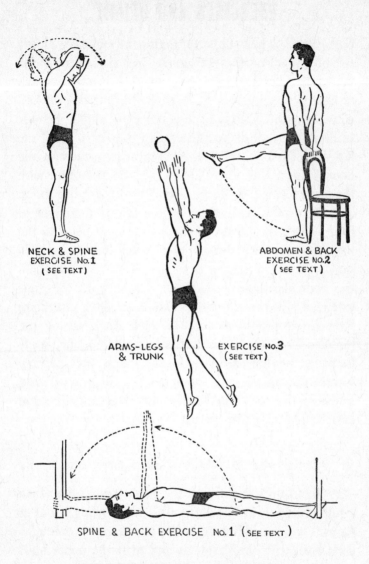

NECK & SPINE
EXERCISE No.1
(SEE TEXT)

ABDOMEN & BACK
EXERCISE No.2
(SEE TEXT)

ARMS-LEGS
& TRUNK

EXERCISE No.3
(SEE TEXT)

SPINE & BACK EXERCISE No.1 (SEE TEXT)

STRETCHING   EXERCISES

torso three or four times toward the right as if trying to turn farther in that direction, rocking the body against the tension of the abdominal and back muscles. Return to the starting point. Duplicate the movement toward the other side, and alternate six or seven times.

2. Stand erect with the feet together, hands on hips, and head and shoulders back. Keeping the upper body straight, turn abruptly to the right and bend the right knee while sliding the left leg, with stiff knee, back along the floor as far as it will go. Return to the starting position and do the same with the other leg. Continue this alternately until tired.

3. Pick out several imaginary spots on the ceiling and, one after the other, leap toward them with both arms outstretched and the head back as if trying to grasp them in the hands; try at each leap to stiffen the legs and arch the back before coming back to the floor. Continue this until some weariness is felt. The same thing may be done with a large, light ball, or better, an inflated toy balloon, tossing it into the air and leaping after it in the above manner while it is still out of reach.

V. EXERCISES STRETCHING THE ENTIRE BODY

1. Make a loop of heavy rope (or a heavy strap sufficiently long will serve) of such size that when it is passed beneath the balls of the feet while standing the hands will just be able to grasp it by stooping the shoulders a trifle. Assume this position and pull up

strongly on the rope, tensing all the muscles of the body in the effort. When the muscles are all tight, increase the stress by slowly rising on the toes as far as feasible without slacking off with the arms. After holding this position for a few seconds relax and repeat the movement until tired. As the rope beneath the toes may throw one off balance, one may easily arrange a short, stout piece of board on which to stand with screw-eyes or ring-bolts on either side of the feet to which the rope may be attached. Or stand on an old chair and pass the rope beneath the seat.

2. Stand with the legs somewhat astride. Raise the arms up straight above the head and in a slow, smooth, continuous motion bring them forward and downward while bending the body and touch the toes with the finger tips. Return to the upright posture, lower the arms to the sides, and relax. Repeat the exercise four to six times. At first it may not be possible to touch the toes with the fingers, but by persisting faithfully in the attempt it will gradually be achieved.

The foregoing exercises offer variety enough for aiding whatever increase in height is possible by this means. Thoroughness, regularity, and persistence in their practice is what is necessary to add to them for success. A few exercises faithfully performed over a period of time will have far more value than a large number of them done sporadically and at long intervals. Nor is it at all necessary to go through the whole list given above at each of the one or two daily exercise periods. That would require some time and would probably tire a person enough to interfere with his day's work. The average person will very likely find that it suffices if he practices one, or perhaps two, of the breathing exercises thoroughly and from the rest picks a group of exercises by choosing one from each class, making a total of five plus the breathing exercises, and doing them well. After following these for a week or two, he may pick out another similar group, and by thus varying his choice from time to time he can get a large number of different groups that will help keep his interest alive by preventing monotony.

There is also a variety of exercise for increasing the height in which the members and muscles are moved and stretched by means of various machines and contraptions that apply far more stress to them than can be managed by one's own movements. Just what is the benefit of this method is difficult to say, though it is asserted (by the promoters, of course) to be considerable. We shall consider this mode of treatment somewhat further in the next chapter.

12

Devices and Height

WE HAVE previously indicated how man's inherent laziness and gullibility make him an easy prey for the hawkers of fraudulent pills and patent medicines for the correction of short stature, as well as for a vast number of other ills. These traits, coupled with a childlike awed respect for things mechanical, especially when they approach the fantastic in design or purpose, also make him a lavish buyer of an infinitude of contrivances, contraptions, gadgets, and whatnot, allegedly intended for purposes similar to those of the pills, but actually in the great majority of instances not a whit more effective. Just as a man will frequently buy a bright, shining tool that he has neither occasion nor knowledge to use, so will he eagerly purchase, at a substantial price, an "electric belt" for backache, a suction cup for baldness, or a "magnetic blanket" for rheumatism, when that same money put into doctor's fees and the same effort put into regular, intelligent care of his malady would result in some real benefit.

It is doubtful that there is any field, great or small, of human ills and defects that has not to some extent been invaded by the quacks with their patent medicines and mechanical devices. It is probable that throughout the year more money pours into the coffers of these charlatans than flows through the channels of legitimate medicine. It is wise never to resort to any of these, regardless of how good they look, without first asking the opinion of a trained doctor.

While the field of stature increase by its very nature lends itself less readily to the activities of the quacks, it is nevertheless by no means free of them and both the pill peddlers and gadget vendors draw an attractive revenue from it.

Devices for increasing the height may conveniently be grouped into three general classes according to the manner in which they achieve, or attempt to achieve, their purpose:

1. *Illusion.* Some devices make no attempt to affect the individual's actual stature, but only to bring about an *appearance* of greater height. This they may do in a number of ways. It may be done by special built-up shoes that raise a person's heels one to several inches from the ground. Or it may be by the cut and pattern of the clothing so fashioned as to make a person appear taller. Or his surroundings, furnishings, and the like may be designed for the same effect. These illusory methods of

DEVICES AND HEIGHT

height increase will be taken up further in chapters 14 and 17.

2. *Posture*. The importance of posture for the person who would have his stature appear at its best has already been mentioned and the subject will be discussed more fully in chapter 13. There are some devices that take advantage of this fact and attempt to work some improvement in stature by forcing the user to assume a better posture. These, of course, take the form of some sort of body, shoulder, or spine brace.

3. *Stretching*. It has been pointed out in the chapter before this that much of the benefit of height-increasing exercises derives from the stretching they induce in the joints, spine, and supporting muscles. The largest number of height-increasing devices are based on this principle and they attempt in various manners to bring about such stretching by mechanical means and also more forcefully and to a greater degree than can be done by ordinary exercise.

The fundamental fallacy of these devices for stature improvement should by now be apparent, and the same holds for devices intended for any bodily defect. In themselves, of course, they can be of no efficacy, but can operate only through employing or applying some agency that may have power in the desired direction. In the present case, as we have just seen, they may be designed to utilize any of three main agencies; namely, illusion, posture correction, or stretching. Now, these methods all have their value and are discussed elsewhere in this

book quite apart from devices. Consequently, any benefit derived from the use of one of these devices derives
from the agency it employs and not primarily from the
device applying it, and conversely no device can be more
effective than the agency it exploits. The conclusion is
simple and obvious. If stature is increased through the
agency rather than the device and the agency may readily
be applied without the mediation of the device, money
spent on even the best of such devices represents a
wholly uncalled for expenditure. And there are many
devices that apply an effective agency very inefficiently
or not at all.

The arrangements for improving posture by mechanical means are almost self-explanatory. It may be a simple
harness of cloth, elastic, or leather straps that fits across
the back and around the shoulders. It may be a tight,
all-encompassing elastic or canvas jacket that laces snugly
about the hips and upper body. Or it may be a rigid steel
and leather brace that straps on and holds the body as in
a vise. But the purpose of them all is to force back the
shoulders, straighten the spine, and make the body be
carried more erectly over the hips. Most of these braces
do bring about a better posture *while they are in place,*
but the improvement is purely artificial and temporary,
not real and permanent as is desirable. The body can be
held in almost any position by binding it there. What is
really wanted is so to strengthen and train the muscles
that they will naturally and without external aid induce
a proper carriage in the body. Any doctor will agree that

the surest manner of weakening a muscle and rendering it useless is by bracing and holding the part it supports so that the muscular support is no longer required, and the best way of strengthening it is by exercising it and consciously and regularly prompting it to perform its neglected duty. Therefore, instead of bringing about the posture improvement that these braces apparently do they really are an enemy to it, for they not only forestall improvement along correct lines, but they also bring about additional weakness of the muscles involved and constantly aggravate the original condition. The longer such braces are worn, the more difficult will it be to dispense with them and the harder will it be to effect proper postural improvement.

All the above remarks, be it understood, are directed only at braces intended for posture correction in otherwise healthy persons. They do not apply to medical braces that are worn to support injured or diseased organs or members whose musculature has become inadequate. This is quite another matter and such braces are often both necessary and helpful. The matter of posture and stature will be further studied in the next chapter.

The stature-increasing devices that make use of the principle of stretching the joints and muscles are of two main sorts: those that merely fasten to the body and stretch it by brute force and those that induce the body to make movements and take postures that will accomplish this stretching. In the latter they put the body mechanically through various exercises that differ not a great deal from those outlined in the preceding chapter, save that they cause them to be done with greater vigor and stress.

Devices of the former sort may consist of arrangements for applying a pull of any desired intensity to the body by any of a variety of mechanical means. Or they may simply be accommodations for holding or suspending the body in such a manner that its own weight supplies the pulling force. An example of the first kind is a couchlike arrangement (selling under the name "Pandiculator") upon which the person lies in such a manner that padded upright stops come in his armpits and his feet fall into a holding contrivance on an extensible portion of the couch. A rachet lever is at the side, within easy reach of the hand, and by operating this the extensible portion holding the feet is made to move outwardly and thus exert a pull on the body which is held from sliding by the armpit stops. Some models also have a similar extensible section at the other end with bands for holding the head around and under the jaw, thus enabling a pull to be applied directly to the whole length of the spine from head to foot. Though we all shudder at the barbarity of the legendary bed of Procrustes, people pay many dollars each year for contraptions of this nature.

Of the second variety of "stretcher" mentioned above —those utilizing the body's own weight for the pulling force—there are some different modifications available, but all work in one manner or another by holding up the upper part of the body and allowing the rest of it to pull downward. Suspension is an early mode of treatment and was fairly popular in the old days of medicine. The theory behind it was that some disorders being traceable to one or another of the many important nerve centers in the spine, suspension of the patient would tend to elongate the spine, relieve pressure or distortion of these centers, and so eliminate the trouble. A common piece of equipment of the old-time doctor was the Sayres apparatus, a sort of stout jacket which strapped about the patient's upper body and by which he was hanged.

Among devices of this nature that have been most notorious in recent years was the Glover height-increasing "halter" that was exposed by the federal authorities as a fraud. It consisted of canvas bands, sewed together so as to fit about the head like a halter, fastened to ropes for attaching it to an overhead beam at a variable height from the floor. Included were two hand grips also on ropes for suspending from the ceiling. The mode of operation was to fasten the head in the halter and have it adjusted so that the feet could barely touch the floor, causing the body to hang by the neck and exert a pull along the length of the spine. The hand grips were to be used to relieve the strain when it became too great. The device was manufactured for about 75 cents and sold for $8.50. Fantastic as the whole notion appears, there were enough gullible people to enable the promoters to clear much money before they were stopped by the authorities.

DEVICES AND HEIGHT

Less barbaric in design but much the same in principle are the devices which fasten to the wall or ceiling and furnish a support from which one may hang or swing by the hands, the weight of the body exerting a pull on the spine as in the previous instance. One such gadget (the "Rota" by trade name) supplies nothing more than a short bar fastened to the wall (at a variable height from the floor) and inclined upward from it, adjustable to various horizontal angles with the wall. It is used by fixing it at a height just within the person's standing reach, who then grasps it and, leaving his feet in one position on the floor, swings his hips outwardly and about in different directions, thus at one time pulling on the spine and subjecting it to a varying curvature that constitutes an exercise for it and the adjacent muscles. This device, according to its advertising, will not only increase the height, but it will also "flood the body with abundant nerve energy," take years off the age, improve the eyesight, relieve constipation, eliminate colds, and bestow a number of other great benefits to ailing mankind.

It is not our purpose to dispute the place or value of spinal or muscular stretching and exercise in height-increasing attempts. Our point is only that every bit as much benefit may be obtained without the use of any elaborate, expensive apparatus, either by the exercises given in the chapter following, or by hanging and swinging from a cheap homemade bar or from any beam or pipe that will support the weight.

120

DEVICES AND HEIGHT

In connection with stature increase by stretching, this is as good a place as any to mention a surgical operation perfected by Dr. Alvia Brockway, of Los Angeles, for remedying a shortness in one leg, usually the result of infantile paralysis or tuberculosis of the hip. He operates on the lower leg. This has two bones: the large tibia and the small fibula. The former he cuts halfway through at a right angle, continues the cut lengthwise down the bone for the distance of the desired elongation, then finishes the cut to the other side of the bone again at a right angle, making a sort of Z-shaped cut with the midportion running up the center line of the bone. The fibula he cuts across on a long slant. Pins are inserted in the bones above and below the cuts and, after the flesh has healed around them, turnbuckles are fastened to them which are so adjusted as to bring about a stretching of 1/25 to 1/20 of an inch per day until the desired length is obtained. The tendons are also cut in the same Z fashion, pulled to the new length at one time, and stitched in place. The various small muscles, blood vessels, and nerves adjust themselves without attention in the course of the gradual stretching. It is asserted that no pain is experienced during the stretching. After five to eight months the turnbuckles and pins are removed and the leg is ready for use. Three inches is the maximum elongation possible by this method. Dr. Brockway has done at least 75 of these operations and he declares they were 90 per cent successful. He unhesitatingly states that in the hands of competent surgeons it is both safe and practical when done below the knee. The muscles of the thigh are too tough and resistant to stretching to make it practicable there.

A natural question is: Why not apply this operation to both legs and thus effect a definite increase in stature? It is a logical possibility, but one that to date hasn't received any encouragement from Dr. Brockway. He has turned down some fat fees offered him for such work by short men. He regards his operation in a serious light, as one deserved only by unfortunates burdened with the great handicap of legs badly disparate in length, and he will not consider its use merely to satisfy personal vanity. However, the time may well come when other less scrupulous surgeons will perfect themselves in the same technique.

13

Posture and Height

CORRECT posture is well worthy of striving for from almost any conceivable angle, from setting off one's clothing better to aiding in the relief of constipation. In the field of height increase it has a twofold importance. First of all, proper posture "unfolds" such stature as one already has and gives it its best height and appearance. If one is slouched over, not only may the top of his head actually be inches closer to the ground than it would otherwise be, but also the drooping, bedraggled aspect of his figure will make even this curtailed stature appear still smaller. Conversely, an upright, alert carriage will of itself make a short person appear taller than he really is. Secondly, good posture is important in that it will contribute greatly to general health by encouraging proper respiration and lung action, by promoting circulation, causing the internal organs to be held as and where they should be and thus enabling the physiological functions to go on more freely. In itself this constitutes a form of exercise for the supporting muscles of the body, which will tend to abet and supplement any other measures that are being made in the direction of height increase.

Good posture is always essential, but from the standpoint of stature it is especially so during the youthful, growing period of life. If during this time the body is habitually carried with the head thrust slackly forward and the shoulders hunched, the chest is cramped and respiration and other internal functions are restricted. Moreover, excess weight is thrown on the spine, with the result that the vertebrae are forced together and compress the cartilaginous cushions between them (inhibiting their expansion, which is an essential factor in growth). Thus are growth, development, and general health much impaired. Wise parents who wish their offspring to attain their best stature (as well as for a number of other significant reasons) will therefore watch and correct their children's posture most carefully. Further, if the habit of correct posture is drilled into a person during his early childhood, it will usually remain with him throughout life without much additional effort.

Now it must not be comfortably presumed that, while admitting the truth of all the foregoing, bad posture and its evil effects are so remote from oneself and one's family as to be little cause for great concern. Just the opposite is the case. Careful and extensive studies indicate that fully 75 per cent of our American youth are afflicted with definitely improper posture. Hence, it is a matter immediate enough to deserve the attention of all of us.

Naturally, no discussion of good posture can long continue without outlining some specifications for it. This has already very concisely been done in a report of the Subcommittee on Body Mechanics of the White House Conference, and we can do no better than to quote the requirements there set forth:

(a) The head with the "chin in," i. e., pulled back until its point is nearly over the sternal notch, is balanced above the shoulders, hips and ankles.

(b) The thorax with the costal angle wide is poised in such a position that the sternum becomes that part of the body farthest forward.

(c) The lower abdomen is held "in" and "flat."

(d) The lower extremities are so aligned with the trunk and head that the lower ends of the femurs and the upper ends of the tibias oppose each other in such a manner as to support the super incumbent body weight with the minimum amount of muscular exertion or tonus.

(e) Good body mechanics [or posture] does not obtain unless the balance of the muscles of the lower extremities is favorable to weight bearing lines which will protect the joint mechanisms of the feet.

This, while entirely good and adequate, is somewhat general and technical in phrasing. We consequently may find some more particular and applicable advice in the "Ten Commandments of Good Posture" as drawn up

POSTURE AND HEIGHT

by Philip Lewin in *Hygeia*, a publication of the American Medical Association:

1. Stand tall.
2. Sit tall.
3. Walk tall and "chesty" with weight transmitted to the balls of your feet.
4. Draw in your abdomen, pulling it back and up.
5. Keep your shoulders square and high but not hunched.
6. Pull your chin straight back toward your collar button.
7. Flatten the hollow of your back by rolling your pelvis down and back.
8. Separate your shoulders from your hips as far as possible.
9. Lie tall and flat. Sleep tall.
10. Think tall.

The next question logically to present itself is: How am I to tell whether my posture is good or bad? To meet this difficulty, Jane Priestly, in an article in *Hygeia*, describes three tests that one may apply to himself in order to determine this matter:

"First . . . try the back-to-the-wall test. Stand against a wall with your heels three or four inches away from it, and with the back of your head, your shoulders and your hips touching it. If your back is properly shaped there will be just room enough for some one to put a

POSTURE AND HEIGHT

hand between the small of your back and the wall. If your back is too flat it will go against the wall almost all the way.

"The second test will tell you where and whether you're out of line. Stand as straight as you can in a doorway, with your back against the corner of the jamb and pull the door toward you until it touches you. If it touches your chin or nose first, your head and neck are too far forward. If it bumps against your stomach, your pelvis is tilted at the wrong angle, and you're probably hollow chested. Now pull yourself up until you occupy as little space as possible. This is correct posture and the door will probably touch your chest first.

"For the third test you will need a three-panel mirror. Stand in front of the mirror and assume the best posture you know. Now look at yourself. Are your feet parallel? Do your ankles turn in? See whether your hips are in line with each other and whether your shoulders are the same height. Your arms should hang loosely, slightly bent, so that your hands are a little to the front.

"Now fix the mirror so that without moving your head you can see yourself in profile. If you are standing as you should the tip of your ear, the point of your shoulder, your elbow and your ankle bone should be exactly in line."

The first step in correcting posture is to learn instinctively to avoid practices that foster bad posture. Generally speaking, these will be any sort of activity, position, or habit that tends to hold the body in a strained, un-

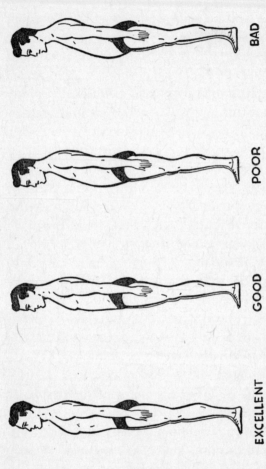

EXCELLENT   GOOD   POOR   BAD

STANDARDS of POSTURE

natural attitude for long periods of time or at frequent intervals. Thus, for example, hours spent sitting in uncomfortable, cramped seats that are unfavorable to a proper sitting posture, long standing with the whole weight on one foot, habitually carrying heavy burdens with the same arm, driving for lengthy periods with one arm elevated high in the window of the car, and similar practices will work to destroy good posture and encourage in its place an unnatural and unhealthful carriage. One must strive constantly to avoid such habits and to conquer any of them he may have fallen into.

As for more positive manners in which faulty posture may be remedied, there is still some disagreement among authorities as to the proper approach. Dr. S. U. Lawton, speaking in New York in 1939 before a conference on posture and body mechanics, took exception to the usual conception of posture as a problem only of bones, muscles, and ligaments. Its fundamental approach, he declared, should be through the entire nervous system and it should be regarded as a dynamic problem involving the whole person. The customary method of treating posture by exercises for specific parts of the body to correct specific defects he claimed to be wrong. Instead, measures should be taken for the good of the whole body. He further stated that the problems of different individuals and of different build vary and require treatments not all of the same kind. Most variables affecting posture, he asserted, are unconscious and outside the control of the will. The approach to correcting posture, therefore, should be through the setting up of remedial conditioned reflexes and must be indirect in nature.

All of which is saying much the same thing we have been insisting upon right along. Merely forcing oneself to assume a correct posture before a mirror for a minute or two morning and evening is certainly not enough for our purpose. Good posture has not been gained so long as it is a matter of conscious effort. What is needed is to have it become habitual, a thing maintained quite unconsciously the majority of time. Regardless of what else may be demanded, two things are certainly requisite: the muscles must be strengthened so they are capable of holding the body properly and they must be trained to keep the body in a correct position at all times naturally and of their own accord. Despite objections that may be raised, it seems quite reasonable that exercise will be at least helpful in bringing this about.

Consciously forcing the body to assume a good posture as frequently and as long as can be managed should therefore aid in training the muscles and impressing their proper position upon them. This can be greatly abetted by exercise which not only will help in the muscle training, but also will increase their elasticity and tone and render them more susceptible to it. Almost any of the exercises already described in chapter 11 will prove of some value in this direction, particularly the breathing exercises. In addition, we shall here outline some other exercises that may be found of benefit in remedying certain special postural defects. These exercises are subject to the same general rules as laid down in the above-mentioned chapter.

Exercises for Improving Posture

1. *For correcting round shoulders.* Stand up as straight as possible. Clasp the hands behind the back, just over the small of the back, and roll the shoulders upward and backward as far as can be managed, keeping the head up and pulling back hard with the elbows. Relax and repeat eight to ten times.

2. *Another for correcting round shoulders.* Sit on a bench or stool without a back. Clasp the hands behind the head and hold the elbows back as far as they will go. Stretch out the whole upper body while extending the arms, hands clasped, above the head, taking care to keep them back as far as can be done. Return to first position, relax, and repeat six to eight times.

3. *For correcting an excessively curved back.* Stand with the back to the wall, the heels three or four inches from it, the back of the head, the shoulders, and the hips touching it. By contracting the muscles of the abdomen and pelvis, force the small of the back firmly against the wall. Relax and repeat. After each third or fourth time walk a few steps away from the wall while holding the back in the straightened position, return, and relax. Continue until tiredness is felt.

4. *For correcting an excessively flat back.* A firm, flat table capable of supporting the weight is needed. Place

the upper body on the table face downward so that the edge comes under the hips and the legs hang down. Place the hands under the chin and keep the neck straight and the elbows out toward the sides. By the use of the back muscles only, raise the legs and head at the same time as high as can be managed, trying to arch the back. Relax and repeat until weariness is felt. At first this will probably not go very well as the muscles will not be strong enough, but gradually as they develop, the head, back, and legs will be able to assume a smooth curve. This had best be practiced cautiously at first, else there will be extreme soreness of the unused muscles.

5. *For lifting the chest and flattening the waist.* Stand with the back to the wall, heels about six inches from it. Press the entire length of the spine, including the waist portion, firmly against the wall, holding the stomach in the whole time. Keeping the elbows down, place the finger tips on the shoulders. Press the elbows against the wall and raise the chest. Then, keeping the elbows tight to the wall, straighten the arms until the back of the hands press the wall and then slowly raise the arms to shoulder height, maintaining a pressure against the wall with all the above-mentioned points. Return slowly to the original position, relax, and repeat the entire exercise five or six times.

In the previous chapter on devices for increasing height there have already been mentioned braces of various sorts for holding the body forcibly in a better posture. One

POSTURE AND HEIGHT

might ask why these are not of benefit since we have just above recommended the regular holding of the body as it should be as a good means of aiding improvement of its carriage. The answer is that by holding the body properly without external aid the muscles are gradually strengthened and trained to do their part in maintaining correct posture, just as the muscles of the arm may be trained by long practice to the expert use of some tool. Whereas if the body is held by a brace that does the work certain muscles should be doing, these muscles lie laxly unused against this support, grow gradually weaker and more negligent of their duty, and the brace, instead of remedying the condition, constantly aggravates it and ends by becoming indispensable.

14

Clothes and Height

THERE is an oft-repeated current phrase to the effect that "Clothes make the man" and there is a great deal of truth in the statement, at least so far as concerns the external man. We may add two words to the above: "Clothes make the man appear taller" and obtain a declaration equally valid and much more pertinent to our present subject.

Naturally, clothing is a matter for consideration with the young, growing person. We have already pointed out how wrong clothing worn during childhood and adolescence—tight, heavy, binding, posture-warping garments—may greatly interfere with and retard growth and development so that the person will not attain the stature that might otherwise be his. But it is not this that is referred to in this chapter. What we are here interested in is the fact that by the proper and intelligent choice and design of the clothing a person may be made to appear appreciably taller whereas by actual measure he has not gained the smallest fraction of an inch in height. Of course, clothing may also be handled so as to make the tall person appear shorter, the stout person thinner, etc., but at the moment we are interested only in what it will do for stature.

Patience, constant attention to details, intelligence, and experimentation so as to get the combination of elements best suited to individual needs are the requisites for success in this matter of dressing for greater stature effect. But while to some extent this will be a separate problem for each man, there are nevertheless a number of fundamental rules governing the matter that must always be observed if the fullest effect is to be achieved. The most important of these are briefly as follows:

1. Always stress the vertical. Emphasize the up and down lines of your costume, both in its cut and in the pattern of the cloth.

2. Minimize the horizontal. This, too, applies both to cut and pattern.

3. Keep the vertical lines as long and as unbroken as possible. Avoid cross lines in the pattern of the cloth; have the vertical lines smooth and straight, not zigzag or curved back and forth.

4. Avoid broadness as much as possible. Fullness about the waist in the cut of the coat or trousers is bad. Double-breasted coats are too ample for a short, heavy man. Nor is fullness in the trouser legs or the sleeves desirable. If the trousers taper a bit toward the ankle it will be

found to help. In sports this same care should be exercised. Beware of plus-fours with a broad plaid design; instead, wear neat-fitting riding breeches, or the like, of a dark, uniform color. And in the cloth pattern do not let even the long, vertical lines get too broad, but keep them narrow or pin stripe. The only exception to this rule is the shoulders. A certain broadness there will aid the illusion of height and manliness of figure, but even this must not be overdone lest the effect be grotesque.

5. Keep the waistline as high as possible without creating an unusual effect. This will give additional apparent leg length. If a belt is worn, be sure to have it narrow, as a wide belt will draw attention to the raised waistline and, by so cutting one's length in two thereby, will work against the illusion of height. Suspenders are still better than even a narrow belt (that is, of course, when they show), for not only is the horizontal line thus eliminated, but the suspenders also help the vertical-line effect.

6. Have the trousers as long as possible and their cuffs narrow. This will aid the appearance of greater leg length. However, have the sleeves no longer than necessary, for if the arms are made to appear long the legs will by contrast with them appear shorter.

7. Wear a hat of some height in the crown. This will add as definitely to apparent stature as will high heels. But do not overdo it lest it attract attention and thus destroy the effect. And do not permit the brim to be too wide as this will surely dwarf one. Avoid going bareheaded or wearing caps or berets.

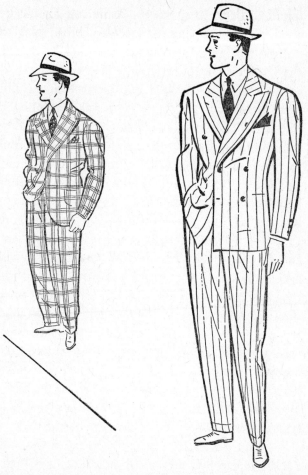

The short-and-thin type can very easily be made to look taller and heavier by proper clothes. He should wear well-proportioned double-breasted suits to suggest width. The patterns should always be hairline, vertical stripes for height, spaced narrowly, not widely. Above all, noisy patterns and extreme lines should be avoided.

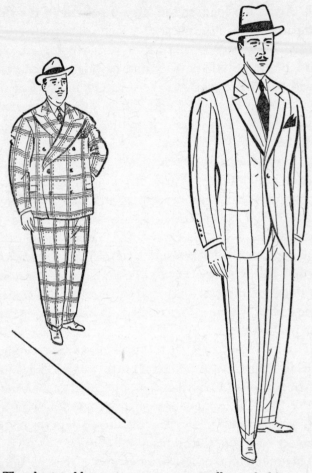

The short-and-heavy type can appear taller and thinner
without much difficulty if the proper clothes are selected.
He should wear only single-breasted suits, and the
patterns should be restricted to subtle, vertical-line
stripes. The worst kind of suit for this type is the double-
breasted with bold patterns like plaids.

CLOTHES AND HEIGHT

8. Avoid too loud or too large a pattern in the shirt and particularly in the necktie. A solid color, thin vertical stripes, or a very small pattern is advisable for the shirt. If the necktie is of a solid or predominant color it will contribute much to the vertical-line effect of the whole. Avoid the "dirty shirt hiders," those excessively broad cravats; keep them as narrow as is in keeping with the rest of the costume.

9. Do not wear large ornaments, jewelry, or accessory articles of clothing. Avoid large, flashing fobs and charms, great lapel pins or insignia, and monstrous finger rings. Do not be smothered in too ample a muffler or overcoat collar. Do not be dwarfed by enormous patch pockets. Have the pockets and lapels as high as practical. Do not have the overcoat too voluminous or too long. Do not have the coat buttons too large and have them placed a bit lower than is customary. Do not wear narrow, long-pointed shoes.

It is important that all these elements be combined tactfully into a consistent, harmonious whole. They must not be permitted to clash or fight one another. Nor must any of them be overdone or out of proportion with the rest, as this would draw the conscious attention of the beholder to it and thus destroy the illusion.

There are some other manners and means of aiding the impression of greater height, which, not falling under the head of clothing, will be found described in chapter 17. If the information there and in the present chapter is adroitly applied and utilized to supplement the increase in stature to be obtained by following the other methods detailed in this book, the short man will soon be able to achieve a noteworthy improvement of his condition.

Our book is concerned chiefly with the stature problems of men as tallness is to them a much more important matter than to women. Naturally, the height-increasing measures previously outlined may be employed by women as readily as by men. And even the present chapter, though it has discussed men's clothing, is applicable in its basic principles to women's dress also. All that has been said about the stress on smooth, unbroken, vertical lines—the avoidance of horizontal lines, the elimination of broadness in the pattern and fullness in the cut, and the use of a high waistline and hats of small width—applies equally to the apparel of both sexes. Dresses should be worn rather than suits to avoid the break in the length. Skirts should be long and without much flare at the bottom. There should be no broad belts—better, none at all. Dresses that are tailored to fit the waist snugly without a belt are excellent for short women. Jackets and capes should be short, no more than waist length at most. Detail of pattern in the material should be confined to the bodice—this will aid the effect of longer legs. Avoid color breaks in the costume, as this will detract from the length. Even the stockings had best be of a shade comparable to the rest of the clothing. Wear small, snug furs, not great, dangling, muffling ones. And observe what has been said above about large ornaments and accessories. Above all, do not allow yourself to be dwarfed by a huge valiselike handbag.

15

Weight and Height

THOUGH we have throughout this book been stressing stature almost exclusively, we must not allow to grow a conception of it as a single, isolated physical characteristic with no relation to or dependence upon other bodily dimensions. A man may be his full six feet tall and still be very much a freak by reason of great disproportion of his other measurements. And conversely a much shorter but well-proportioned man may present a far more attractive figure because of the harmony of his lines. Consequently, it must never be forgotten that height is but one of several external manners in which growth and development manifest themselves.

One of the most obvious correlatives of height is the general bulk of the body as a whole since this represents the result of true, three-dimensional growth as contrasted to the unreal unidimensional growth as measured by stature solely. Body bulk is rather difficult to gauge as volume, but as it bears a close relation to weight, the latter may be taken as a convenient estimate of the former. And this is very widely done. The ratio of weight to height furnishes a much-used indication of the degree and normality of bodily development.

But the ratio of weight to height is not the same for all periods of life. And the same applies to the ratio of the rates at which they increase. Dr. H. W. Haggard sums up the situation as follows:

"During growth the percentage increase in weight is greater than the increase in stature. This means that the body fills out as well as elongates, but less than as the cube of the height. The weight per unit of length becomes greater as maturity is approached. Thus the weight of an average boy or girl of seven, 20 kilograms, divided by the height, 11.5 decimeters, gives a value of 1.8; at fourteen years this becomes 3.0; and at maturity the average figure is 4.0. For a young adult a height-weight relation in decimeters and kilograms of 4.0 represents good proportioning of the body; 5.4, obesity; and 3.6, emaciation. These same values given in the relation of inches and pounds are 2.2, 3.0, and 1.9 respectively."

However, the height-weight relation must not be regarded as a close, tight function of growth, any small deviation from which is to be viewed as abnormal. Indeed, there is always room for some doubt as to just what may constitute the "normal" value in this ratio. Individual peculiarities may affect it somewhat without any especial disorder being indicated by the discrepancy.

WEIGHT AND HEIGHT

Elaborate height-weight tables have been drawn up that indicate a weight that is suitable for any given height and vice versa. But these should not be taken too seriously in an exact sense as they after all only represent the averages struck from the figures offered by a large number of apparently healthy and normal persons of varied sizes. Consequently, these tables must be used with intelligence. However, if a person's height-weight ratio varies from that given by an accepted table by more than 10 per cent it may usually be taken as an indication of the presence of some disorder in the functions of growth in that person.

Another factor in gauging height is age, as has already been discussed in chapter 8, but this is of a kind with weight in that its relation with stature cannot be regarded at best as more than approximate. Indeed, it is commonly conceded by authorities to be impossible to draw up any airtight connection between age, weight, and height as there are too many variables and individual peculiarities and circumstances that may enter the picture and influence the figures without its being possible truly to say that they affect the normality of the case.

As a matter of fact, despite the general acceptance of the height-weight ratio as a measure of development, Dr. Mary L. Boillin, a research worker at Teachers College, Columbia University, found that height is one of the least dependable factors in determining weight. Naturally, it would be of no more value for an estimate in the reverse direction. Dr. Boillin found several other body dimensions to be in closer consonance with weight than is height, the best of all being the depth of the chest. The degree or percentage of importance of various dimensions in determining weight she found to be as follows:

Shoulder width, 9 per cent;

Height, 16 per cent;

Width of hips, 20 per cent;

Width of chest, 23 per cent;

Depth of chest, 32 per cent.

According to this, weight bears a poorer relation to but one body measurement than it does to height. Naturally, these figures are not above dispute. Nevertheless, if intelligently used, tables of height in relation to weight, as well as to age, may be of considerable service in forming some estimate of the degree of one's growth and the need of or advisability of an attempt to increase the stature so as to bring it up to the normal average. Therefore, in the next chapter we reproduce two such tables, again cautioning against interpreting them too literally.

16

Tables of Heights

HEIGHT AND WEIGHT TABLE FOR MEN

Height with shoes—weight with clothes

Height	15-19 Years Lbs.	20-24 Years Lbs.	25-29 Years Lbs.	30-34 Years Lbs.	35-39 Years Lbs.	40-44 Years Lbs.	45-49 Years Lbs.	50 Years and Over Lbs.
5 ft. 0 in.	113	119	124	127	129	132	134	135
5 ft. 1 in.	115	121	126	129	131	134	136	137
5 ft. 2 in.	118	124	128	131	133	136	138	139
5 ft. 3 in.	121	127	131	134	136	139	141	142
5 ft. 4 in.	124	131	134	137	140	142	144	145
5 ft. 5 in.	128	135	138	141	144	146	148	149
5 ft. 6 in.	132	139	142	145	148	150	152	153
5 ft. 7 in.	136	142	146	149	152	154	156	157
5 ft. 8 in.	140	146	150	154	157	159	161	162
5 ft. 9 in.	144	150	154	158	162	164	166	167
5 ft. 10 in.	148	154	158	163	167	169	171	172
5 ft. 11 in.	153	158	163	168	172	175	177	178
6 ft. 0 in.	158	163	169	174	178	181	183	184

TABLES OF HEIGHT

HEIGHT AND WEIGHT TABLE FOR WOMEN

Height with shoes—weight with clothes

Height	15-19 Years Lbs.	20-24 Years Lbs.	25-29 Years Lbs.	30-34 Years Lbs.	35-39 Years Lbs.	40-44 Years Lbs.	45-49 Years Lbs.	50 Years and Over Lbs.
4 ft. 8 in.	104	107	110	113	116	120	123	125
4 ft. 9 in.	106	109	112	115	118	122	125	127
4 ft. 10 in.	108	111	114	117	120	124	127	129
4 ft. 11 in.	110	113	116	119	122	126	129	131
5 ft. 0 in.	112	115	118	121	124	128	131	133
5 ft. 1 in.	114	117	120	123	126	130	133	135
5 ft. 2 in.	117	120	122	125	129	133	136	138
5 ft. 3 in.	120	123	125	128	132	136	139	141
5 ft. 4 in.	123	126	129	132	136	139	142	144
5 ft. 5 in.	126	129	132	136	140	143	146	148
5 ft. 6 in.	130	133	136	140	144	147	151	152
5 ft. 7 in.	134	137	140	144	148	151	155	157
5 ft. 8 in.	138	141	144	148	152	155	159	162

17

Stature Aids

WE HAVE already in earlier chapters gone into the various methods of aiding short stature as much as is practicable. All the direct and indirect measures for achieving this end have been discussed according to type —from exercise, posture, diet, etc., to devices and clothing. There yet remain a few means that may be made to contribute to our purpose which do not fall into any of the categories already treated, and these we shall consider briefly in the present chapter.

One of the surest ways to raise the head higher from the ground is to stand on something. That is to say, by putting extra material in the shoes so as to elevate the feet higher from the ground one may readily be made to seem taller. High heels will serve the purpose very nicely, and this is a method much in vogue with women, though perhaps for reasons of style as much as for tallness. However, high heels throw one's feet, and even the entire body, into an unnatural, strained position. Attempts to remedy this by building up the soles of the shoes result in footwear so clumsy and unwieldy in appearance as to destroy whatever advantage the added height may give. Besides, high heels look effeminate and grotesque on a man, and men are more in need of stature aid than are women.

There have been many endeavors in the history of the world to aid stature by means of specially constructed, thick-bottomed shoes, but it is only recently that they have achieved any great degree of satisfaction. Naturally, the ideal shoe of this sort must effect a considerable elevation of the feet from the ground while presenting an external appearance no different from that of an ordinary shoe. There is available one make of such a shoe ("Staturaids," made by Joseph Burger of New York City) that manages this very nicely. It builds up the heel, and to some extent the sole, *inside* the shoe, bringing the leather of the uppers down on the outside so that only a normal amount of sole-edge and heel is open to view. The price of these shoes is perhaps a trifle high ($14.50 to $19.50, depending on the amount of elevation), but they are well constructed, being handmade, of good leather, and will probably wear longer and look better than cheaper machine-made shoes, to say nothing of the value of their height-increasing effect. They offer any desired elevation in stature up to $2\frac{1}{4}$ inches in the regular models, and one may have even more in special designs. Undoubtedly, such shoes offer one of the surest and most immediate means of making oneself appear taller, and when combined with proper clothing can do very much for even the shortest of persons.

Though short women are at less of a disadvantage than men, they too may now obtain shoes made in this same fashion, though the lift possible is not as great for them as for the men. Their shoes being of daintier, flimsier, more open construction, it is not possible to hide as much material under their feet. However, a lift of as much as an inch has been very successfully obtained (by Dan Palter, of Palter de Liso, New York City) by running extra material under the sole and heel while tapering it (mainly from the outside) to paper thinness under the arch where the uppers are open or drop down to the sole. This scheme permits its application to the daintiest of evening shoes as well as to street or sports wear of sturdier construction.

In his own home, the short person can do a great deal to aid the illusion of tallness merely by the exercise of a little care and ingenuity in the selection and arrangement of the furnishings. Since the furnishings supply the background against which one's stature is projected and measured by the eye of the observer, avoidance of any great contrasts between the two will leave the eye to presume a normal height in the other person. Also, by scaling down the size of the various ordinary articles of furniture that are instinctively taken to be of a standard size, the short person is made to appear taller in relation to them. If one can afford it, he should have his wall panels, chairs, tables, draperies, and the like all made to dimensions somewhat below the usual; they would work a distinct heightening effect on him while in their presence. In the office the same thing could be done with the desk, chairs, cabinets, etc. If normal-size furniture is desired because of guests who will use it, much the same effect of smallness (with the lesser contrast so beneficial to the short man) may be gained by a proper choice of design. Slender, straight lines, thin legs, flat and non-ornate surfaces of a color tending toward the dark, chair backs of open construction that are not too high, cabinets that are less tall than customary, and rounded corners and delicate lines throughout will make furniture appear smaller than it really is and consequently will make the person using it or near it appear taller. Large, bulky, or massive pieces of furniture should be avoided as completely as possible. And hanging pictures, mirrors, and other wall decorations lower than is commonly done will greatly help the person in the room.

Finally, in the field of stature aids, there is the matter of behavior, mannerisms, and personal conduct of the short person. In general, avoid a too youthful appearance. Youthfulness is instinctively associated with immaturity and smallness. Proper clothing will help much in this—dark colors, conservative pattern and cut, etc. Chapter 14 treats the clothing problem more fully. A mustache, too, will help combat a youthful appearance, but it must not be overdone—huge "handle-bars" will dwarf a short man and be worse than none at all. A certain amount of

STATURE AIDS

aggressiveness is necessary in a small man to overcome the negativeness of his size, but it must not be carried too far lest it become mere ridiculous "cockiness." Eyeglasses (if worn) should be carefully chosen: the big goggle-eyed, heavy rimmed ones are bad for a short person; the small, light rimless variety is infinitely better. Be seated in company as much as possible because differences in height are less noticeable in this position. However, do not sit in great commodious armchairs that will seem to swallow you as a trifling morsel. When standing, do not be too near large or tall pieces of furniture or under high pictures, wall hangings or fixtures. Try to stand in front of low, horizontal lines and surfaces, near small, low pieces of furniture. Do not stand in front of high, vertical lines, near high curtains, tall cabinets, or in or before high windows or doorways. When standing talking to other persons, do not stand too close to them or facing them too directly. The closer you are to the other the more aware is he of your shortness. Do not carry any large object that will tend to emphasize your own smallness. Newspapers folded only once (roll them up tightly), large magazines or books (carry the pocket size), large, thick canes, huge, voluminous umbrellas, big trunklike valises, etc., should all be avoided. Do not smoke oversize cigars or a huge pipe; it is better to stick to cigarettes in public. Do not stand in an obviously strained erect position or keep the shoulders noticeably back. And as for personal conduct, do not strut, boast, or talk too loudly, and above all do not pick fights.

18

Psychological Aids

WE HAVE in the antecedent chapters studied the factors governing growth and stature and the ways and means in which they may be affected and stimulated in persons in which they have been retarded to the extent of being a handicap or source of embarrassment. Much can be done by the short person to remedy his condition, as a perusal of the preceding chapters will demonstrate, but we cannot in truth claim that *everything* can be done by these measures and that the short man can be made the full equal of the six-footer in many respects. In any field, corrective measures as a rule only *relieve* a condition or defect but do not do away with it entirely, and to this the methods of stature increase are no exception.

Therefore, while striving to do all he can to help his height, the small man should early reconcile himself never to be truly a big man in a physical sense and to learn to adopt a reasonable, sensible attitude toward his stature. To be sure, to be short is often a disadvantage and a hindrance, but certainly it is no tragic cause for shame and ceaseless agonizing. Undue concern over shortness stems usually more from reasons of vanity than from any other, and the better this is understood the more endurable will one's condition become. Vanity makes one think his stature should match what he fondly imagines to be his otherwise "big" personality. Vanity makes one think that everyone notices his shortness, whereas in fact most people are like oneself and are much too concerned with themselves to give much heed to the characteristics of others. Besides, like it or not, he can rarely do more than correct it partially, so he had as well accept cheerfully what he will have to accept anyway and get some enjoyment from life. Further, constant preoccupation with and touchiness on one's shortness will only serve to draw the attention of others to it, whereas otherwise they would probably never notice it at all.

Furthermore, there is no real reason for a small man to feel inadequate or out of things. There is too much evidence pointing in the opposite direction. Tallness and bigness, past reasonable limits, is very often not at all desirable, and may in fact frequently be an inconvenience and expense. For one thing, from a purely physiological viewpoint, excessive growth seems often to take place at the expense of other bodily attributes and faculties. Records clearly show that giants are weak and incompetent—usually their minds are poor, they can hardly move their own bodies, they have no endurance and tire easily, and are generally impotent. A lesson may be learned from the prehistoric dinosaurs mentioned earlier: their one great faculty was to grow bigger and ever bigger until finally they became so large that they could not get food enough to subsist and so perished from the earth.

So the wise person will not wish to grow too fast or too large after all. It has been noted by a number of investigators that an accelerated rate of growth will ofttimes bring about a premature aging. We have already remarked in a previous chapter that a diet which promotes growth seems to have a definitely deleterious effect upon longevity. And perhaps the tall are not such a happy, fortunate race after all. Drs. A. A. Piney and P. B. Skells, two well-known London physicians, agree that the majority of suicides are long-legged persons; that they are more likely than the short-legged to become depressed, act on impulse, and thus in many cases take their lives. It appears that tallness and bigness exact many penalties that the short and small are spared.

It stands to reason that the short man will wish to do everything possible for his height, but once this is done he will not, if wise, allow the matter constantly to prey upon his mind or oppress his spirit. The psychological approach to the problem of short stature is as important as any of the others discussed in this volume. What most unhappy small men lack in even greater degree than they do height is a sense of humor broad enough to enable them to make sport of their own condition before anyone else has opportunity to do so, and thus magically destroy the power of all present to hurt them. Treat your physical condition in a jovial, joking manner just as a large man might do with his, an artist with his talent, or a bachelor with his so-called freedom. Your shortness is one of your attributes just as the other qualities are of the other persons; there is nothing either criminal or praiseworthy in it. It is merely a physical fact to be faced and is no more occasion for shame than is the unfortunate fact that it may happen to rain on the day you arrange a picnic for your friends.

Learn to make capital of your condition. It will give your conversation a distinct turn, aid in covering over many a dull spot, and give you the reputation of a welcome enlivening element in company, an accomplishment that will endear you to people far more than a few extra inches of height. Train your mind to be alert and your tongue to be quick at repartee so that if big, thick-witted fellows try to goad you about your size you are able to parry their gibes with pertinent remarks about whatever obvious failings they have. This will be found fairly easy, for there is generally a great lack of imagination in the modes of attack in "kidding" a short person. "Shorty," "Half-pint," "Sawed-off," and the like are fair examples of the unoriginality of the nicknames commonly employed. Thus, one may soon work up a neat set of responses for each possibility and have it ever ready to confound the teaser. And never forget that in any sort of contest the sympathy of the crowd is always with the smaller man. Even when the large man is wholly in the right the attitude usually is "Pick on somebody your size!"

Learn to think and act tall. Judge yourself by qualities other than your height—your intelligence, loyalty, honesty, expertness in some craft or art, etc. And learn to realize that these really make the man and could not necessarily be improved by being taller. By not always having your mind preoccupied by your smallness you will soon become as unconscious of it as are the people around you. Always remember that, in common with all physical and most physiological characteristics, there is possible great variation in stature without passing the bounds of normality. An adult may range in height from 4 feet 1 inch to 6 feet 6¾ inches without being a freak or abnormal in any way. Anyone below this minimum is a midget or above this maximum, a giant. But the very great majority will fall well between the limits and are therefore—save by foolish, artificial standards—normal men as to height.

It must never be forgotten that shortness is by no means a bar to greatness. Indeed, as we have pointed out previously, the short man has a much better chance of greatness than the man of average stature. And history certainly bears this out. Frederick the Great, Epictetus the Roman philosopher, Blake the poet, Horace the ancient Roman poet, Alexander the conqueror, Archimedes the first experimental scientist, Erasmus, Linnaeus the great botanist, Mozart, Chopin, Spinoza, Gibbon, Balzac, Heine, Milton, Michelangelo, and of course Napoleon, as well as many other celebrated figures of the past, were all definitely below average height, and many of them very much so. Among internationally known persons of the present day we find: Mayor La Guardia of New York, 5 feet 4 inches; Billy Rose, the famous producer, 5 feet 5 inches; Adolph Zukor, the great movie producer, 5 feet 2 inches; Mussolini, 5 feet 5 inches; Irving Berlin, the composer, 5 feet 4 inches. And this list could be made much, much longer. It often seems that short persons may really be more fortunate than those of average size as they are driven to greatness and achievement in other fields as a means of compensation.

In our present machine age, which is becoming more and more mechanized by the day, size in a person is coming to count for less and less. Expertness, alertness, resourcefulness, quickness, agility—all qualities that the small man ordinarily possesses to a much greater extent than the large man—are coming into increasing demand. And with the growing tendency toward compactness and economy of space, his very smallness in itself is becoming a desirable attribute and an asset in earning a livelihood. We are living in an age of shrinking dimensions—from candid cameras and midget radios, through Austin automobiles, to digest magazines and tablets in which the vitamin content of several full meals is concentrated to the size of a pea—and the small man should more than ever be coming into his own.

And there are many practical advantages accruing to the short man. His food and clothing will cost him less, since he requires a lesser quantity. The restaurant meal that would be woefully insufficient for a big man will be quite adequate for him without the expense of additional purchases. Large-size clothing costs all out of proportion with the extra material needed. And wherever space is at a premium the short man is at a distinct advantage. In theaters, public conveyances, hotel beds, camp cots, Pullman berths, all places where the large man will be miserably cramped, the small man will be quite at ease. And the bumps from low doors, ceilings, beams, and pipes he is spared! For him a trip in a trailer can be a truly enjoyable vacation, not merely the more or less exasperating experience it offers the tall man. And the short man, being more agile by nature and capable of slipping through small openings, will find it much simpler to avoid and escape accidents of all sorts, which is no trivial matter in our present machine age. Indeed, insurance companies have found the small man to be much the better risk.

The small woman has even less reason for self-pity. All the above listed advantages belong to her also. Her saving on clothing will be still greater than the man's, for the much cheaper misses', or even girls', sizes will fit her admirably. The small woman satisfies the romantic ideal much oftener than the large, sturdy woman. Her "petiteness" gives her an added charm and men rush in to "protect" the helpless creature. She can wear becomingly extremes of style and color in her clothing and get away with things a tall woman would never dare try.

PSYCHOLOGICAL AIDS

And, finally, the short woman always appears younger than the tall woman (because of an instinctive connection in the mind between smallness and youth) and is thus granted an attribute that women prize most highly.

All of which is not to say that the average man would not prefer to be tall and robust for, say what you will, he would. But if this cannot be, there is certainly small cause for wailing and despair, as our above remarks should by now have demonstrated. The small man has no real cause to be pitied or to pity himself; on many scores he may even be envied. And, judging by results, one would say that he seems usually well able to take care of himself and is rarely seen to come out at the short end of things.